Research and Evaluation in Community, Health and Social Care Settings

How can we develop a comprehensive understanding of the research process in community, health and social care settings?

Covering all stages of the research process, from funding to dissemination, this book considers the views of funders, researchers, communities and policy makers. Drawing on practical examples and relevant international literature, it sheds light on issues that can arise in the process and presents solutions and strategies to deal with a range of challenges.

Organised around a series of themes that capture the essential elements of the research process including covering framing research in theory, commissioning and designing research, utilisation of findings and knowledge transfer, this book provides practical guidance for those involved in child welfare and education, nursing and clinical practices, community studies and the social sciences. It will be a key resource for all those who are interested in developing their understanding of the research and evaluation process in these areas.

Suzanne Guerin is an associate professor in research design and analysis with the UCD School of Psychology at University College Dublin. Her research interests include applied health and wellbeing, and applied research and evaluation. Suzanne has developed significant expertise in these areas and as a result is involved in a number of projects nationally and internationally. She is Deputy Director of the UCD Centre for Disability Studies and a member of the All Ireland Institute of Hospice and Palliative Care (AIIHPC) Palliative Care Research Network.

Nóirín Hayes is a developmental psychologist with particular interest is early child development and learning, curriculum and pedagogy and children's rights. She is the author of a number of books, reports and research articles on early childhood education, practice and policy including *Early Years Practice: Getting it Right from the Start* (2013, Gill and Macmillan) and co-author of *Introducing Bronfenbrenner* (2017, Routledge). She has served on a number of government advisory and working groups and commissions, and is a founder member of the Children's Rights Alliance and an honorary member of OMEP international.

Sinéad McNally is an assistant professor in psychology at the Institute of Education at Dublin City University. She holds a BA in French and psychology (Trinity College Dublin) and a PhD in psychology (Trinity College Dublin). She is experienced in conducting and managing research in the academic and voluntary sectors in Ireland, and specialises in children's earliest experiences and the factors that impact on children's early health, language and social-emotional development.

Routledge Advances in Health and Social Policy

For a full list of titles in this series, please visit https://www.routledge.com/Routledge-Advances-in-Health-and-Social-Policy/book-series/RAHSP

Titles in this series

M-Health in Developing Countries
Design and Implementation Perspectives on Using Mobiles in Healthcare
Arul Chib

Planning Later Life
Bioethics and Public Health in Ageing Societies
Edited by Mark Schweda, Larissa Pfaller, Kai Brauer, Frank Adloff and Silke Schicktanz

Effective Interventions for Unemployed Young People in Europe
Social Innovation or Paradigm Shift?
Edited by Tomas Sirovatka and Henk Spies

Social Research in Health and Illness
Case-Based Approaches
Constantinos N. Phellas and Costas S. Constantinou

Forthcoming titles

Ethnic Identity and US Immigration Policy Reform
American Citizenship and Belonging amongst Hispanic Immigrants
Maria del Mar Farina

Research and Evaluation in Community, Health and Social Care Settings
Experiences from Practice
Edited by Suzanne Guerin, Nóirín Hayes and Sinéad McNally

Research and Evaluation in Community, Health and Social Care Settings

Experiences from Practice

Edited by
Suzanne Guerin, Nóirín Hayes and Sinéad McNally

Routledge
Taylor & Francis Group
LONDON AND NEW YORK

First published 2018 by Routledge

2 Park Square, Milton Park, Abingdon, Oxfordshire OX14 4RN
52 Vanderbilt Avenue, New York, NY 10017

Routledge is an imprint of the Taylor & Francis Group, an informa business

First issued in paperback 2019

British Library Cataloguing in Publication Data
A catalogue record for this book is available from the British Library

Library of Congress Cataloging in Publication Data
Names: Guerin, Suzanne, editor. | Hayes, Nóirín, editor. | McNally, Sinéad, editor.
Title: Research and evaluation in community, health and social care settings : experiences from practice / edited by Suzanne Guerin, Nóirín Hayes and Sinéad McNally.
Description: Abingdon, Oxon ; New York, NY : Routledge, 2018. | Series: Routledge advances in health and social policy | Includes bibliographical references and index.
Identifiers: LCCN 2017027049 | ISBN 9781138308275 (hardback) | ISBN 9781315142920 (ebook)
Subjects: LCSH: Community-based social services–Research–Methodology. | Community health services–Research–Methodology. | Public welfare.
Classification: LCC HV11 .R39626 2018 | DDC 361.0072–dc23
LC record available at https://lccn.loc.gov/2017027049

ISBN: 978-1-138-30827-5 (hbk)
ISBN: 978-0-367-43105-1 (pbk)

Typeset in Times New Roman
by Taylor & Francis Books

Contents

Illustrations

Figure

Table

Boxes

REPP project team

The Research Evaluation Policy and Practice (REPP) Project Group brings together researchers, practitioners/service providers and policy makers from a range of disciplines, all of whom are involved in commissioning, conducting and/or disseminating research with children, families and communities in a variety of settings throughout the island of Ireland. The REPP project was funded by The Atlantic Philanthropies and managed by the Childhood Development Initiative. The REPP project team oversaw the development of the proposal and assisted in the identification of authors. The members of the team are (in alphabetical order):

- Prof. Catherine Comiskey – School of Nursing & Midwifery, The University of Dublin, Trinity College Dublin
- Dr Gemma Cox – *youngballymun*, Dublin
- Dr Orla Doyle – UCD Geary Institute & UCD School of Economics, University College Dublin
- Dr Jane Gray – Department of Sociology & National Institute for Regional and Spatial Analyis, Maynooth University
- Associate Prof. Suzanne Guerin **(Chair)** – UCD School of Psychology & UCD Centre for Disability Studies, University College Dublin
- Prof. Nóirín Hayes – School of Education, The University of Dublin, Trinity College Dublin
- Dr Claire Hickey – Centre for Effective Services and (previously) Barnardos Ireland
- Prof. Sinéad McGilloway – Centre for Mental Health and Community Research, Department of Psychology, National University of Ireland, Maynooth
- Dr Sinéad McNally – Institute of Education, Dublin City University
- Dr Tara Murphy – Formally Tallaght West Childhood Development Initiative (CDI) and All Ireland Institute of Hospice and Palliative Care (AIIHPC)
- Ms Marian Quinn – Tallaght West Childhood Development Initiative

Contributors

Gail Birkbeck, is the (former) head of Strategic Learning & Evaluation (EuroAfrica) at The Atlantic Philanthropies, an international foundation. She is a research psychologist working in the field of evaluation and research for the past 27 years, both nationally and internationally. For the last 13 years, Gail was responsible for evaluation strategy and implementation on the island of Ireland and South Africa at The Atlantic Philanthropies, the largest foundation to ever end its grant making. This entailed commissioning and managing research and evaluation studies as well as disseminating findings for maximum use and impact.

Catherine Comiskey is a professor in health care modeling at Trinity College, Dublin and has over 20 years' research experience and has a particular interest in the design, implementation and execution of evaluations of treatment and intervention programmes with a view to providing research-based evidence for policy and service delivery decisions. She also has a particular interest in using bio-mathematical and statistical models to identify key factors that improve outcomes from interventions.

Pat Dolan is the UNESCO Chair in Children, Youth and Civic Engagement at the National University of Ireland, Galway. He is joint founder and Director of the UNESCO Child and Family Research Centre, where he also directs the MA in family support studies. Prof Dolan has over 20 years working with families as a practitioner, service manager and academic, completing research in areas such as adolescents' perceived mental health, resilience and support networks.

Maresa Duignan is the assistant chief inspector for early years education in the Department of Education and Skills. Formerly she was an early years education specialist advising the Ministers for Education and Skills and Children and Youth Affairs on a range of national policies, including the development of national strategies to address issues related to funding and governance of the early years sector, evaluation and monitoring of provision and practice and inclusion of children with disabilities. She also represents Ireland on European Commission and OECD working groups on early childhood education and care.

Jane Gray is a professor of sociology at Maynooth University. Her published research centres on questions relating to families, households and social change. She is a research associate in the Maynooth University Social Sciences Institute, where she is the programme leader for the Irish Qualitative Data Archive (www.maynoothuniversity.ie/iqda), and principal investigator on the Irish government funded Digital Repository of Ireland (www.dri.ie). Her most recent book is a co-authored textbook (with Ruth Geraghty and David Ralph), *Family Rhythms: Changing Textures of Family Life in Ireland*, published by Manchester University Press.

Claire Hickey is a senior project specialist with the Centre for Effective Services in Dublin, where she manages the ABC Evaluation. She previously worked as a senior research manager with Barnardos, were she was responsible for a range of activities including implementing and managing Barnardos research and evaluation programme, analysing secondary data sources, promoting quality research and knowledge transfer and participating in external research advisory groups.

Grainne Hickey is the research programme manager of the ENRICH study in the Centre for Mental Health and Community Research at Maynooth University. She studied for her BA in psychology at Trinity College Dublin and completed a PhD in 2009, also at TCD. In 2009 she moved to Maynooth to join the then Mental Health and Social Research Unit as a postdoctoral researcher. In 2013 she was part of a group which won a 5-year HRB grant to evaluate wraparound interventions for vulnerable children and families in Ireland – ENRICH.

Siobhán Keegan is a developmental psychologist with a special interest in how young children learn and develop, particularly within the context of early years settings. Her PhD research was a longitudinal study focusing on the age-16 educational outcomes of a sample of children, taking into account the contexts of home, school and preschool. She works as a coordinator with Better Start Early Years Quality Development Service, which provides mentoring support to early years services to develop and sustain quality. She has over 10 years' experience leading research projects and evaluations with children, families, schools and early years settings, and has worked as a research consultant, nationally and internationally. Her interests include child and adolescent development, quality in ECEC settings and mentoring theory and practice.

Gemma Kiernan is an associate professor in psychotherapy with the School of Nursing and Human Sciences at Dublin City University. She has previously worked in health, education and social services and is a registered psychologist and counselling psychologist with the Psychological Society of Ireland. Gemma's research explores aspects of children's psychosocial health and development in the areas of illness, disability and loss.

Sinéad McGilloway is professor in mental health care research and well-being and founding director of the *Centre for Mental Health and Community*

Research (formerly the Mental Health and Social Research Unit), Department of Psychology, National University of Ireland, Maynooth. She is a research innovator and leader, educationalist, public health/community psychologist and health services researcher, with many years' experience in undertaking policy and practice-relevant health and social research focusing, in particular, on child and adult mental health and wellbeing in community contexts, and service evaluation.

Jennie Milnes is a clinical psychologist with experience of conducting research in clinical and community-based settings. She has coordinated longitudinal research to examine the efficacy of novel psychological treatments for drug and alcohol misuse, and for mood and other mental health difficulties. She has conducted hundreds of research interviews on socially sensitive topics and her blend of clinical skills, academic rigour, and a warm and empathic manner have contributed to her successes in this. In 2016 she was awarded the Áine O'Callaghan award by the Health Service Executive and Trinity College Dublin in recognition of her clinical and research skills working with children and families.

Mark Morgan is Cregan Professor of Education and Psychology at the Institute of Education, St Patrick's Campus at Dublin City University, and has previously served as co-director of Growing Up in Ireland longitudinal study. He studied at the London School of Economics and Stanford University. His research interests have included the evaluation of prevention programmes and educational disadvantage. In 2010, he was awarded the president's prize for research by Dublin City University.

Tara Murphy recently commenced a career break after working for over five years as programme manager research with the All Ireland Institute of Hospice and Palliative Care (AIIHPC). A significant element of her role within the Institute was leading on the all-Ireland Palliative Care Research Network as well as on a large interdisciplinary research capacity building programme. Previous to that Tara worked as research and evaluation manager at the Tallaght West Childhood Development Initiative (CDI) for over four years where she managed the implementation of an extensive evaluation and research programme in health, education and community development. Tara has a BA in microbiology (Trinity College Dublin), BSc in psychology (Open University) and a PhD (Trinity College Dublin). Her doctoral research examined the support needs of parents of children on the autistic spectrum from the diagnosis onwards.

Elizabeth Nixon is an assistant professor in developmental psychology at the School of Psychology, Trinity College Dublin. Elizabeth holds a BA and an MLit in psychology from University College Dublin and a PhD from Trinity College Dublin. She is co-director of the Infant and Child Research Lab at TCD, where she investigates parent-child interactions and their relation to children's development. She was co-investigator on Phase 1 of the Growing Up in Ireland, the national longitudinal study of children, and is currently the TCD lead investigator for Phase 2 (2015–2019).

Morgan O'Brien is a lecturer in the Department of Humanities at the Institute of Technology Carlow. He has previously worked as research project coordinator in the Mental Health and Social Research Unit (Maynooth University) and the Centre for Youth Research and Development (Maynooth University).

Aileen O'Carroll is the policy manager at the Digital Repository of Ireland (DRI). She is based in the Maynooth University Social Science Institute (MUSSI), where she manages the Irish Qualitative Data Archive (IQDA). This role involves the development and implementation of standards for deposit and access to qualitative data (text based, audio and visual) in line with emerging international and EU standards. She additionally advises researchers on best practice in managing and archiving research projects, both to ensure that ethical commitments are met and that the data gathered is of the highest standard to facilitate optimal re-use by a variety of audiences. In the field of digital data her research interests are concerned with research methods, ethics and privacy and research data management.

Eylin Palamaro-Munsell is a lecturer in the Psychological Sciences Department at Northern Arizona University, having previously taught at Arizona State University. Before this she was the research coordinator of the evaluation of Preparing for Life at University College Dublin's Geary Institute. She holds a PhD in community psychology and an MA in clinical community psychology from the University of North Carolina Charlotte, with a BA in psychology from the University of Vermont.

Marian Quinn is the CEO of an organisation co-funded by government and philanthropy to design, deliver and evaluate the effectiveness of a range of services for children and families and has overseen the commissioning, dissemination and translation of a significant body of research. Marian has previously worked in the Department of Justice, the Health Services Executive and the volunteer sector. She wrote and managed the "Copping on Programme", a national crime prevention initiative, and has published widely in relation to youth crime. She is co-author of *Click Click* (Hachette) and has been central to a number of cross border developments.

Gráinne Smith is a quality specialist with the Childhood Development Initiative, a Dublin organisation working to promote prevention and early intervention. She has been involved in designing and supporting the delivery of a range of evidence-based interventions, working closely with front line practitioners. She currently coordinates an intervention to promote positive parenting for fathers in prisons. Gráinne has a background in children's nursing and holds a Master's in education from NUI Maynooth. She has presented internationally on effective implementation approaches, co-written a number of articles in relation to models of best practice in early intervention speech and language services and has vast experience of translating research into practice.

Foreword

More than ever, children, youth, parents and families need greater capacity to cope, particularly those who experience adversity and ongoing challenges in their lives. So the development and mainstreaming of "promising or proven" preventive initiatives that enable families to thrive is vital. Similarly, we are moving swiftly towards an era where the relationship between associated social research and evaluation of programmes and interventions that underpin such developments can no longer be unread, static written reports, but must provide active usable evidence. This also has to include sharing evidence around what work best for families, but equally important, how and why it works for them. With this in mind, and in the context of a major philanthropic investment in Irish services, programmes and communities, the production of this book is particularly welcome and timely.

In a very concise fashion, the editors and contributors have brought together research and evaluation learning into what are well-articulated helpful practice lessons and policy relevant messages. As director of one of the research centres that have been heavily involved and invested in this philanthropic initiative in Ireland, I am particularly delighted that the book very honestly explores and shares the challenges and tensions of the real world research relationship between evaluators and service providers.

Just as good relationships are the key to all successful family support practices, one of the lessons to be found here in this volume is that the same rule applies to researchers and practitioners. Throughout the chapters the blended mixture of theory (knowing of), policy (knowing to) and practice (knowing how) becomes a unique composite of knowledge and wisdom in working with children, youth, families and their communities in the context of underpinning and associated research evaluation policy and practice. This is invaluable to all stakeholders from academia, to service managers and more importantly those working at the coal-face of practice. However, the ultimate positive legacy here leans towards better systems and practices that positively affect the lives of children and families in need. This is in all our interest.

Professor Pat Dolan
UNESCO Chair in Children, Youth and Civic Engagement
UNESCO Child and Family Research Centre
National University of Ireland Galway

Acknowledgements

The REPP Project was funded by The Atlantic Philanthropies and supported by the Irish Department of Children and Youth Affairs. We are grateful for their support with this project.

Thanks go to the Childhood Development Initiative, who have managed and housed the project since its inception. We are also grateful to the Centre for Effective Services for their input early in the project's development.

Finally, we would also like to recognise the significant contribution of the three Prevention and Early Intervention Programme sites, whose work stimulated much of the learning in this text: The Childhood Development Initiative, Preparing for Life and *youngballymun*. For more information on these programmes visit their websites:

- http://www.twcdi.ie
- http://preparingforlife.ie
- http://www.youngballymun.org/home

Royalties from this publication will be donated to The Society of Saint Vincent de Paul. www.svp.ie

1 Introduction

Suzanne Guerin and Claire Hickey

Introduction

This book aims to serve as a guide for researchers, practitioners, commissioners and consumers of research who are interested in research with children, families and communities conducted in real world contexts. It is the product of a collaboration of individual researchers, practitioners and policymakers actively involved in these areas of research in Ireland. Given the aim of the book, the task of this introduction is to provide a context for the later chapters by describing the background to, and nature of, these changes. The international practice of collaboration between philanthropy and government to address pertinent research, practice and policy issues has contributed to a significant amount of research worldwide. In Ireland, the provision of funding and leadership by The Atlantic Philanthropies (AP) and the Irish government has coincided with a greater emphasis on multidisciplinary thinking and collaboration between researchers, practitioners and policymakers across settings. This chapter sets the Irish experience in the international context. In addition, this chapter will describe the aims of the Research, Evaluation, Policy and Practice (REPP) Project, which has produced this text, and how it grew out of this context. There are two key elements of the context to be considered: the international literature on research and practice with children, families and communities, and the specific context of Ireland as a setting that has undergone significant change economically and socially during its recent history.

The international context

The translation of scientific or research evidence into policy and practice is a key component in the development of effective education, health and welfare systems. It is a complex process involving concepts such as knowledge transfer, evidence-based practice and policy and implementation science – concepts which are woven throughout this text. However, the process of conducting and communicating meaningful research in a way that ensures it has the desired impact on policy and practice remains challenging, on both a national and international basis. This challenge exists across many disciplines, including child welfare, education, nursing, clinical practice, community studies and other areas of the social sciences (Ward et al., 2012; Wiggins, Austerberry & Ward, 2012). However, developments in research have contributed towards more effective practice in this area.

Cooperation between researchers and practitioners is common, with the ultimate aim of providing an insight into applied issues. This cooperation is exemplified by the growth of community-based participatory research (CBPR). Minkler and Wallerstein (2008, p. 6) cite the W.K. Kellog Foundation's Community Health Scholar programme definition of CBPR as

> [Involving] all partners in the research process and recognizes the unique strengths that each brings. [It] begins with a research topic of importance to the community with the aim of combining knowledge and action for social change to improve community health and eliminate health disparities.

The edited text by Minkler and Wallerstein reflects on the foundations of the approach and the challenges and contribution of CBPR before concluding on the contribution of this approach to creating meaningful change. The emphasis on greater community involvement reflects the key principles of CBPR, which Wallerstein and Duran (2006) describe as recently emerged research paradigm. While the authors represented in this text may not formally frame their work as CBPR specifically, it is possible to identify different aspects of its key principles in a number of the case studies. Building on this, it is important to recognize the theoretical context of CBPR. Chapter 2, which follows, identifies two theoretical frameworks commonly applied to CBPR. The first is the ecological systems approach (Nelson & Prilleltensky, 2010), which recognizes the complex, multidirectional interactions evident in these settings. The second relevant theory considered in Chapter 2 is the empowerment framework, a central principle of which is improving individuals lives by empowering them (Cattaneo & Chapman, 2010).

Considering the application of the CBPR approach to research, Minkler, Blackwell, Thompson and Tamir (2003) discuss the role that philanthropy and government play in encouraging and supporting community-based research in public health. Roob and Bradach (2009) stress the benefits of these two domains collaborating to address research, practice and policy issues in the lives of children, families and communities. The published literature has considered issues of governmental, non-governmental and philanthropic funding of programmes to promote development in many parts of the world, and indeed there is consideration of public–private partnership in this area. However, there appears to be less consideration of the potential for effective partnership between philanthropy and government. The current text is grounded in the learning that has been sparked in part by the collaboration in Ireland between The Atlantic Philanthropies and the Irish government (www.atlanticphilanthropies.org/evaluations/evaluation-prevention-and-early-inter

vention-programme-ireland-and-northern-ireland). The specifics of this collaboration will be considered later in this Introduction.

The topic of partnership more broadly in research has been raised in many disciplines. One area where there has been some debate regarding partnership is public health. Israel, Schulz, Parker and Becker (1998), in a useful review of partnership approaches to community-based research, focus on inequalities in health status. Interestingly the authors note that individuals working in this area have called for a number of key developments to support understanding and implementation in this area including:

- increased attention to the complex issues that compromise the health of people living in marginalized communities;
- more integration of research and practice;
- greater community involvement and control, for example, through partnerships among academic, health practice, and community organizations;
- increased sensitivity to and competence in working within diverse cultures;
- expanded use of both qualitative and quantitative research methods.

(p. 174)

Many of these points will be reflected implicitly and explicitly as themes throughout this text. For example, the chapters present the lessons learned from engagement with a range of community actors, highlighting the challenge of working with diverse groups. Dissecting this call in more detail highlights some of the benefits and challenges of conducting authentic and effective research that has the potential to change policy and practice and contribute to the general development, health and wellbeing of target groups. Clearly the growth of multidisciplinary applied research into issues affecting individuals and communities is the result of increased interest in these complex issues. The final point made by Israel and colleagues captures a key element of this volume – the need for a broad toolbox of methods when working in real world settings. The challenge of involving multiple stakeholders, actors and perspectives in partnership driven research is, we would argue, best met by an openness to adapt the research methods available to the demands of the context. This requires a sense of the demands of effective evidence but an ability to balance this with the nuances of a less controlled context in terms of research. Again, the studies discussed in this volume span the full range of methodological approaches available in the health and social sciences and focus on the process of conducting research.

However, the real success of this multidisciplinary and collaborative research approach is the impact that it has in terms of implementation in policy and practice. The growth of implementation science (e.g. Eccles et al., 2009; Proctor et al., 2009), perhaps represented by the development and success of the open-access journal *Implementation Science*, reflects the increased interest in and commitment to the integration of research and practice. The chapters in this volume draw on a wide range of applied case studies, each of which focuses on different aspects of child, family and community wellbeing and development. However, central to each case is the intent to contribute to positive outcomes for target groups through the completion and implementation of research in real world settings.

In considering the extent to which research informs policy, terms such as evidence-based policy and evidence-informed policy might suggest a relatively easy movement from research to policy. However, many authors have highlighted the process as challenging (e.g. Young, Ashby, Boaz & Grayson, 2002), with Pawson, Greenhalgh, Harvey and Walshe (2005) referring to it as formidable. Authors also highlight the need for research to lead to practice changes, and Kitson et al. (1998) present a number of models of evidence-based practice. Shediac-Rizkallah and Bone (1998) reflect on the challenges of sustainability, recognizing the need for clear operational definitions of what this means. In addition, Altman (1995) considers the need to develop relationships within real world contexts and design interventions that are relevant beyond the lifespan of the research as ways of promoting longer-term change. However, perhaps it is helpful to consider the difference between sustaining practice changes and mainstreaming them. A distinction may be drawn whereby sustaining change in response to research functions at a more local level and reflects the continuation of the immediate process supported by the research, whereas mainstreaming is about the broader implementation of learning (possibly via higher level policy changes). Another way to distinguish between the two would be to view them as a continuum containing three levels: (i) effecting the actual change and maintaining it at the local level throughout the intervention, (ii) sustaining that change once the researched intervention is no longer being researched and (iii) mainstreaming at a higher level of thought, planning and action – which is critical to sustaining the change at local level. Whatever the definition applied to the desire to achieve change as part of the research process, the projects considered in this volume reflect on this issue in different ways, facing the challenge of both sustaining or maintaining change when evidence supports it, but also responding when the evidence fails to emerge as hoped.

Having reflected on key aspects of the international context for research and evaluation and how it relates to policy and practice, this Introduction now turns to the immediate context within which this text and the overarching REPP project developed. This project is motivated by the desire to capture the significant learning that has taking place in Ireland in the last 15 years, recognizing that Ireland has served and continues to serve as a case study of the parallel growth of research and evaluation and evidence-based practice with children, families and communities.

Learning from the Irish experience

The Irish experience provides valuable learning about the intersection of evidence-informed practice and policy with evaluation and evaluation methods – learning that has emerged from two initiatives implemented over the period 2006–2012. During this period, child and family services, serving children and their families in disadvantaged communities across Ireland, benefitted from investment by government and The Atlantic Philanthropies, through their Disadvantaged Children and Youth Programme. Two different, albeit parallel, programmes of investment were introduced: the Prevention and Early Intervention Programme (PEIP) and the Prevention and Early Intervention Initiative (PEII); the former was jointly funded by the Department of Children and Youth Affairs (DCYA) in the Republic of Ireland and The Atlantic Philanthropies, an international philanthropic foundation, while the latter was an initiative solely funded by The Atlantic Philanthropies and covered the whole island of Ireland. The purpose of both the PEIP and the PEII was to examine and evaluate innovative methods for improving outcomes for children in an integrated way, with a focus on mainstreaming evidence-based programmes. The focus on prevention and early intervention services in the PEII was predicated on an understanding that intervening early in a child's life, or early in the onset of a difficulty, supports the achievement of more positive outcomes for children and their families. This understanding has been supported in many areas of child health and wellbeing including mental health (Kieling et al., 2011), positive parenting (Turner & Sanders, 2006), obesity (Paul et al., 2009) and broader child development outcomes (Wise, da Silva, Webster & Sanson, 2005).

In Ireland, three Dublin-based projects were funded through the PEIP joint initiative: the Tallaght West Childhood Development Initiative (CDI), Preparing for Life and *youngballymun*, all of which feature in this book. Funding of €36 million was provided to PEIP over the lifetime of the initiative (2006–2012) for implementation and evaluation – €18 million provided by the government (via the Department of Children and Youth Affairs) and €18 million by The Atlantic Philanthropies. The PEII, supported by The Atlantic Philanthropies, funded a range of other prevention and early intervention initiatives across the island of Ireland, delivered through a variety of predominantly community and voluntary organizations and some public sector providers, too many to list here but including Barnardos, Archways, Foróige, Fatima Regeneration and the Health Service Executive. The use of evidence-based interventions and the requirement to rigorously evaluate efforts were central features of both the PEIP and PEII, and so began an unprecedented process, in Irish terms, of innovation and evaluation in social services for children and their families. Thirty-nine organizations, delivering more than fifty interventions, were involved in the PEIP and PEII; it is estimated that throughout the island of Ireland, 90,000 children, 24,000 parents or caregivers and 4,000 professionals participated in or benefitted from the PEIP and PEII (Rochford et al., 2014). Twenty-five of the 52 interventions were the subject of randomized controlled trials or quasi-experimental evaluations, and the remainder were evaluated using a variety of methods and approaches. This publication documents the experiences of the researchers and service providers involved in evaluating some of these 52 interventions.

Both the PEIP and PEII were predicated on the basis that the 'best' evidence would be used to inform the development of the individual projects funded by these two initiatives, and where the evidence did not exist, or was not sufficiently compelling, that rigorous evaluation methods would be employed to enhance the evidence base. While most providers agree that services should be developed on the basis of the best evidence available, there is some debate about what constitutes the 'best' evidence and how this can inform policy and practice (Young et al., 2002). The appropriateness of using narrowly defined terms such as 'evidence-based' practice and policy has been much discussed in the literature; the more inclusive concept of evidence-informed practice, first used in the social sciences by Hargreaves in 1999 (Shlonsky, Noonan, Littell & Montgomery, 2011) in the context of education, is now used more widely in the Irish policy and services context. The use of the terms evidence-informed practice and evidence-informed policy recognize that knowledge can be generated in many different ways; evidence-informed approaches draw on the relevant evidence from policy and research, but also take into account professional judgement and expertise, service users' views and local context (Yost et al., 2014). Many of the interventions described in this volume represent complex community change initiatives – initiatives that are multi-layered and require changes in, and reform of, service delivery and service coordination (as described in Chapter 8). These types of complex community change initiatives do not lend themselves well to the more familiar and traditional approaches to programme evaluation, such as randomized controlled trials (RCTs) or quasi-experimental studies (QES), typically used to provide an evidence base. Thus, relying solely on evidence generated via RCTs or QES could potentially exclude a range of important and valuable learning for policy-makers and service providers. A series of papers commissioned by the Medical Research Council in the UK has placed the RCT, as one design, in the context of a range of research designs that are suitable for the evaluation of complex, in this case, health interventions (Campbell et al., 2000; Craig et al., 2008; Moore et al., 2014). Researchers and other professionals interested in assessing the contribution of social and educational interventions should also draw on these discussions. As noted by Shlonsky et al. (2011), evidence-informed policy or practice suggests that decisions concerning policy and practice are guided by evidence not based solely upon it, an important distinction where programmes or interventions do not lend themselves to the use of rigorous evaluation designs or in circumstances where the potential for investment in rigorous RCTs for social programmes is unlikely, as is the case in Ireland.

As the various chapters of this book demonstrate, the job of evaluating complex community-based initiatives has been long and complicated, although not without its rewards and in many cases not yet finished. The challenges currently facing those who work in the field of prevention and early intervention service provision to children and their families in Ireland are many. As has been widely documented elsewhere, Ireland experienced a deep recession between 2008 and 2014. As part of its efforts to cut the budget deficit and meet commitments made under an EU-IMF bailout, a national recovery plan was agreed for the period 2011–2014 during which a €15 billion fiscal adjustment was undertaken. Two-thirds of the €15 billion budgetary adjustment came from cuts to social and welfare programmes (Dukelow & Considine, 2014; Hick, 2014), and there was a 13 per cent drop in expenditure on social protection from the 2010 spending level (Hick, 2014). In this context, both statutory and non-statutory community-based services for children and their families have experienced significant funding cuts, and though the economy continues to recover in Ireland, there is no guarantee that social expenditure will return to pre-recession levels. In this climate, there is a danger that the emphasis in service provision will focus once again on crisis and/or treatment interventions and that prevention and early intervention services will be viewed as a luxury rather than an essential part of the continuum of services available to children in need. We will return to this issue in the conclusion of this text.

While the current economic climate suggests a somewhat uncertain future for the mainstreaming of the types of early intervention and prevention programmes discussed in this book, there are reasons to remain optimistic. *Better Outcomes, Brighter Futures*, the national framework for children and young people, 2014–2020, was published in 2014 (Department of Children and Youth Affairs [DCYA], 2014). The national policy framework establishes prevention and early intervention as a key transformational goal. Government has committed to achieving nine substantive actions over the lifetime of the national framework, a central commitment being to work towards rebalancing resources to place greater emphasis on prevention and earlier intervention across a number of key government departments (Department of Children and Youth Affairs, Department of Health, Department of Education and Skills and Department of Justice) and state agencies (Tusla and the Health Service Executive) (DCYA, 2014). Moreover, the mechanisms and institutional arrangements for the delivery of services to children and their families have also been the subject of change with the establishment of Tusla (Child and Family Agency) in 2013, the first dedicated state agency responsible for child welfare and protection services in the state. Learning from the PEIP and PEII has informed the development of the Area Based Childhood (ABC) Programme, an initiative funded by government and by The Atlantic Philanthropies. The ABC Programme targets investment in evidence-informed interventions to improve the long-term outcomes for children and families living in areas of disadvantage. It aims to break "the cycle of child poverty within areas where it is most deeply entrenched and where children are most disadvantaged, through integrated and effective services and interventions" (DCYA, n.d.). Thirteen communities in the Republic of Ireland are participating in the ABC Programme.

The REPP Project

The changes in Ireland described above, and the associated growth in rigorous research and evaluation, have highlighted the learning and knowledge that have been accumulated by the community of professionals working in communities. The Research Evaluation Policy and Practice (REPP) Project Group brings together a diverse group of researchers and practitioners/service providers from a range of disciplines, all of whom are involved in commissioning, conducting and/or disseminating research with children, families and communities throughout the island of Ireland. The REPP project was set up to reflect on and document the process of researching and evaluating the lives of children and their families. In this, REPP is not a novel endeavour by any means. The volume edited by Connell et al. (1995) documents some of the work of the Roundtable on Comprehensive Community Initiatives for Children and Families and the Steering Committee on Evaluation within that group, which formed the basis for the Aspen Institute's (www.aspeninstitute.org) policy programme. While the project that underpins the current volume does not aspire to the same level of influence as the Aspen Institute, the two programmes share many aims. The principal aim of the REPP initiative is to promote and support the effective and judicious production of research findings to policy and practice through a number of channels. Most of the members of the REPP project are involved to a greater or lesser extent in this work and are committed to maximizing its impact and, in particular, to capturing and documenting the key learning for researchers across different settings. The learning from this period of research and implementation in Ireland has significant relevance for individuals outside the Irish context.

Overview of the content

In each of the following chapters, presented within three sections, the authors draw on their own experience in Ireland and the published literature from other countries to provide others with an insight into the challenges and solutions when researching the lives and experiences of children, families and communities. The authors aim to make the material accessible to a broad range of stakeholders, though some topics will be more relevant to different groups working within the broad area of community, health and social care. Section 1 considers the early phase of research and evaluation, and includes chapters on: theoretical frameworks relevant to research with children, families and communities; the commissioning, procuring and contracting process for evaluation research; the realities of governance in these contexts; and finally reflections on the nature and role of key stakeholders in these activities. Section 2 focuses on the process of conducting research and evaluation in community, health and social sectors. The chapters consider the process of research design, data collection and fieldwork, as well as reflecting on the nature of credible evidence. Section 3 addresses the processes of communicating and disseminating research and evaluation knowledge, with chapters on dissemination of findings to multiple stakeholders and the issue of knowledge exchange, culminating with reflections on the challenges and benefits of archiving data from research in these areas in order to maximize the learning. Finally, the book closes with a reflective conclusion, which draws out the key messages from the REPP project and considers their implications for international learning and practice in research with children, families and communities.

References

Altman, D.G. (1995) 'Sustaining interventions in community systems: On the relationship between researchers and communities', *Health Psychology*, 14(6), pp. 526–536.

Campbell, M., Fitzpatrick, R., Haines, A., Kinmonth, A.L., Sandercock, P., Spiegelhalter, D. & Tyrer, P. (2000) 'Framework for design and evaluation of complex interventions to improve health', *British Medical Journal*, 321, pp. 694–696.

Cattaneo, L.B. & Chapman, A.R. (2010) 'The process of empowerment: A model for use in research and practice', *American Psychologist*, 65, pp. 646–659.

Connell, J.P., Kubisch, A.C., Schorr, L.B. & Weiss, C.H. (1995) *New approaches to evaluating community initiatives: Concepts, methods, and contexts.* Washington, DC: The Aspen Institute.

Craig, P., Dieppe, P., Macintyre, S., Michie, S., Nazareth, I. & Petticrew, M. (2008) 'Developing and evaluating complex interventions: The new Medical Research Council guidance', *British Medical Journal*, 337, pp. 979–983.

Department of Children and Youth Affairs (DCYA) (n.d.) *Area Based Childhood (ABC) programme 2013–2017*. Available from www.dcya.gov.ie/viewdoc.asp?fn=%2Fdocuments%2FNational_Childrens_Advisory_Council_.htm&mn=betq&nID=3&mn=arep4s&nID=1.

Department of Children and Youth Affairs (2014) *Better outcomes brighter futures: The national policy framework for children and young people 2014–2020*. Dublin: The Stationery Office.

Dukelow, F. & Considine, M. (2014) 'Between retrenchment and recalibration: The impact of austerity on the Irish social protection system', *Journal of Sociology & Social Welfare*, XLI(2), pp. 55–72.

Eccles, M.P., Armstrong, D., Baker, R., Cleary, K., Davies, H., Davies, S., Glasziou, P., Ilott, I., Kinmonth, A.L., Leng, G., Logan, S., Marteau, T., Michie, S., Rogers, H., Rycroft-Malone, J. & Sibbald, B. (2009) 'An implementation research agenda', *Implementation Science*, 4, p. 18.

Hick, R. (2014) 'From Celtic Tiger to crisis: Progress, problems and prospects for social security in Ireland', *Social Policy & Administration*, 48(4), pp. 394–412.

Israel, B.A., Schulz, A.J., Parker, E.A. & Becker, A.B. (1998) 'Review of community-based research: Assessing partnership approaches to improve public health', *Annual Review of Public Health*, 19, pp. 173–202.

Kieling, C., Baker-Henningham, H., Belfer, M., Conti, G., Ertem, I., Omigbodun, O., Rohde, L.A., Srinth, S., Ulkuer, N. & Rahman, A. (2011) 'Child and adolescent mental health worldwide: Evidence for action', *The Lancet*, 378(9801), pp. 1515–1525.

Kitson, A., Harvey, G. & McCormack, B. (1998) 'Enabling the implementation of evidence based practice: A conceptual framework', *Quality in Health Care*, 7, pp. 149–158.

Minkler, M. & Wallerstein, N. (2008) *Community-based participatory research for health: From process to outcomes.* 2nd edn. San Francisco, CA: Jossey-Bass.

Minkler, M., Blackwell, A.G., Thompson, M. & Tamir, H. (2003) 'Community-based participatory research: Implications for public health funding', *American Journal of Public Health*, 93(8), pp. 1210–1213.

Moore, G. F., Audrey, S., Barker, M., Bond, L., Bonell, C., Hardeman, W., Moore, L., O'Cathain, A., Tinati, T., Wight, D. & Baird, J. (2014) 'Process evaluation of complex interventions: Medical Research Council guidance', *British Medical Journal*, 350, p. h1258.

Nelson, G. & Prilleltensky, I. (2010) *Community psychology. In pursuit of liberation and well-being*. 2nd edn. New York, NY: Palgrave Macmillan.

Paul, I.M., Bartok, C.J., Downs, D.S., Stifler, C.A., Ventura, A.K. & Birch, L.L. (2009) 'Opportunities for the primary prevention of obesity during infancy', *Advances in Pediatrics*, 56(1), pp. 107–133.

Pawson, R.., Greenhalgh, T., Harvey, G. & Walshe, K. (2005) 'Realist review – A new method of systematic review designed for complex policy interventions', *Journal of Health Services Research & Policy*, 10(1), pp. 21–34.

Proctor, E.K., Landsverk, J., Aarons, G., Chambers, D., Glisson, C. & Mittman, B. (2009) 'Implementation research in mental health services: An emerging science with conceptual, methodological, and training challenges', *Administrative Policy in Mental Health*, 36, pp. 24–34.

Rochford, S., Doherty, N. & Owens, S. (2014) *Prevention and early intervention in children and young people's services: Ten years of learning*. Dublin: Centre for Effective Services.

Roob, N. & Bradach, J.L. (2009) *Scaling what works: Implications for philanthropists, policymakers, and nonprofit leaders.* The Edna McConnell Clark Foundation and The Bridgespan Group.

Shediac-Rizkallah, M.C. & Bone, L.R. (1998) 'Planning for the sustainability of community-based health programs: Conceptual frameworks and future directions for research, practice and policy', *Health Education Research; Theory & Practice*, 13(1), pp. 87–108.

Shlonsky, A., Noonan, E., Littell, J.H. & Montgomery, P. (2011) 'The role of systematic reviews and the Campbell Collaboration in the realisation of evidence-informed practice', *Clinical Social Work Journal*, 39(4), pp. 362–368.

Turner, K.M.T. & Sanders, M.R (2006) 'Dissemination of evidence-based parenting and family support strategies: Learning from the Triple P – Positive Parenting Program system approach', *Aggression and Violent Behaviour*, 11(2), pp. 176–193.

Wallerstein, N.B. & Duran, B. (2006) 'Using community-based participatory research to address health disparities', *Health Promotion Practice*, 7, p. 312.

Ward, V. *et al.* (2012) 'Exploring knowledge exchange: A useful framework for practice and policy', *Social Science and Medicine*, 74(3), pp. 297–304.

Wiggins, M., Austerberry, H. & Ward, H. (2012) *Implementing evidence-based programmes in children's services: Key issues for success.* London: Childhood Wellbeing Research Centre. Available from www.cwrc.ac.uk/resources/documents/DFE-RR245_Main_report.pdf.

Wise, S., da Silva, L., Webster, E. & Sanson, A. (2005) *The efficacy of early childhood interventions.* Australian Institute of Family Studies Research Report No. 14. Melbourne: Australian Institute of Family Studies.

Yost, J., Dobbins, M., Traynor, R., DeCorby, K., Workentine, S. & Greco, L. (2014) 'Tools to support evidence-informed public health decision making', *BMC Public Health*, 14, p. 728.

Young, K., Ashby, D., Boaz, A. & Grayson, L. (2002) 'Social science and the evidence based policy movement', *Social Policy and Society*, 1, pp. 215–224.

2 Framing research in community settings

Elizabeth Nixon and Eylin Palamaro-Munsell

Introduction

The aim of this chapter is to discuss the approaches that frame research in community settings. Inherent within all conceptual and theoretical frameworks that guide research are fundamental assumptions and organizing principles about the phenomenon under investigation (Winegar, 1997). In this chapter, we will consider some of the prevailing assumptions and values underlying models for community research. In the sections that follow we will highlight two common frameworks for community research – the ecological framework and the empowerment framework – and illustrate their application, drawing upon international examples of community research.

Ecological approaches to community research

The essence of ecological approaches is to construct an understanding of the relationships among individuals and the social structures and processes of the groups and communities within which they live and work (Kelly et al., 2000). The principle of an ecological approach was first introduced in the 1960s (Kelly, 1966; Trickett, Kelly & Todd, 1972) and has since become an important paradigm for guiding research and intervention efforts in community settings. A central tenet of the approach is that communities are open systems comprising *different levels* and *interdependent connections* among the levels (Nelson & Prilleltensky, 2010).

The levels of the community eco-system have been usefully conceptualized by Bronfenbrenner (1979, 2005) to include the micro-, meso-, exo- and macro-systems. The first, the micro-system, is any setting in which an individual spends time engaging in activities and interactions. Common examples of micro-systems include home, school, workplace or community group. The meso-system reflects relationships across different micro-systems, for example, the relationship between a child's home life and school life. The exo-system refers to contexts within which individuals are not situated but which nonetheless have an important indirect influence on individuals. An example might be how a partner's stressful work environment influences the quality of the couple relationship, and so indirectly affects the individual's wellbeing. Finally, the macro-system context encompasses any group (culture, subculture or extended social structure) whose members share values or belief systems, resources, challenges, lifestyles, life course options and patterns of social interchange (Bronfenbrenner, 1993; Tudge et al., 2009). Furthermore, "the macrosystem envelops the remaining systems, influencing (and being influenced by) all of them" (Tudge et al., 2009, p. 201). This approach espouses the value of *holism* which reflects the importance of focusing upon the whole person in the context of his or her multiple social and personal relationships and the many varied settings in which he or she might be embedded (Prilleltensky & Nelson, 2009).

All the components of an eco-system are interconnected, and changes in one part of the system will ripple out to affect other parts of the system. This is known as *interdependence*. It is important to note that interdependence includes persons as well as settings: persons affect settings and settings affect persons; persons influence other persons; and one setting can affect another setting (Kingry-Westergaard & Kelly, 1990). Thus, intervention at a community level, through, for example, developing or implementing a new service or reducing the negative impact of environmental or social factors, requires an understanding of current interdependencies between people and the structures in the system, as well as the potential for generating new interdependencies (Kelly et al., 2000).

An ecological approach focuses analysis upon the transactions between persons and systems, as well as an analysis of persons and their inter-relationships within the system, and systems' relationships with other systems. Arising from this perspective, issues and problems faced by individuals (e.g. poverty) can be contextualized across multiple levels of analysis, including characteristics of individuals (e.g. physiological reaction to stress), micro-system contexts (e.g. family support) and macro-level analysis (such as policies that determine the availability of income support).

While the ecological metaphor as it applies to research in community settings has in the main been developed within the field of community psychology, the concepts and principles are not unique to this domain. For example, within the field of human development, Urie Bronfenbrenner's ecological theory (1979) initially gave pride of place to aspects of an individual's context in shaping development, while later formulations of his theory further emphasized the individual's role in their development and the processes that underpinned the connection between the individual and some aspect of the context (Bronfenbrenner & Morris, 2006; Tudge et al., 2009, 2016). Similarly, a systemic approach to understanding families is central in the field of family therapy (Dallos & Draper, 2010). Inherent within family systems theory is the view that the whole family is greater than the sum of its individual family members and that in order to understand the functioning of families, one must understand the interdependent relationships between and among family members (Klein & White, 1996).

Other principles of an ecological approach include *adaptation, cycling of resources* and *succession* (Kelly, 1968; Kelly et al., 2000; Nelson & Prilleltensky, 2010). Adaptation refers to how persons and systems within an eco-system respond to change within the eco-system. Change within an eco-system is not linear, and attempts to change one part of the system will often bring unanticipated side effects on other parts of the system. Adaptation does not refer to passive adjustment, however; rather it refers to active efforts to influence the social structure and processes within a system, while at the same time responding to the demands of the system. Kelly et al. (2000) cite as an example of adaptation how teachers and the school system respond to the changes in the ethnicity of the school population.

Cycling of resources is concerned with how resources within an eco-system are identified, developed and allocated. Indeed, central to the ecological perspective is an endorsement of community resource development and capacity building (Trickett, 2009). Resources can be mobilized within individuals or within systems. Personal resource potentials denote the opportunity for people within a social system to use their particular skills, qualities or knowledge to promote the social competence of other people in the system. When personal resource potentials or social norms to support the development of personal resources are present in a system, other persons can seek out informal ties. A low level of personal resource potential may indicate that barriers in the environment are inhibiting the development of personal resources (Kelly et al., 2000). Social system resources refer to groups, procedures and events that affect the development of social systems. These resources serve to promote the social competence of persons within the system, and include things such as money, information and traditions that facilitate persons' integration within the system. According to Kelly et al. (2000), an ecological perspective assumes that there are many more resources within a system than are perceived to be available, and thus an ecological approach should seek to identify and tap into previously unidentified resources.

Finally, succession denotes adopting a long-term perspective, both with reference to the historical context of a problem and the need for planning for a preferred future (Kelly, 1968). By taking a longitudinal perspective on the eco-system and considering historical forces and factors that feed into the current state of the system, a greater understanding of the barriers and facilitators of change can be achieved (Peirson et al., 2011).

The research process conducted through an ecological lens

Adopting an ecological approach to research within a community setting has implications for the research process. The implications of the ecological approach for the research process are well captured by Trickett (1986, p. 190):

> The spirit of ecologically-based consultation is to contribute the resourcefulness of the host environment by building on locally identified concerns

to create processes which aid in empowering the environment to solve its own problems and plan its own development.

An initial step in conducting an ecologically based inquiry involves gaining an awareness of the eco-system, and initiating relationships with key stakeholders within the community. Related to this, Kelly (1971, 2006) describes the development of an eco-identity on the part of the researcher which refers to a commitment on the part of the researcher to learn about and become involved in the community. Thus, the ecological perspective advocates that the researcher's own identity should be related to the community within which he/she works. This early stage also involves conducting an assessment of the environment, thus providing a basis for understanding the acceptability of the research or the implementation of an intervention or prevention programme (Trickett, Kelly & Vincent, 1985). Part of this assessment process involves appreciating and expressing tolerance for the diversity within the community. Thus, different groups may interact differently with their ecological environment (Trickett, 1996) and community programmes may be designed to target the needs of specific groups within the community. This process also reflects part of a broader process of being responsive to the community context. According to Trickett et al. (1985), this entails appreciating local concerns and commitments and incorporating these into the conceptualization, development, implementation and evaluation of any programme. In practice, this responsiveness to the community context may be manifested in how a specific programme is tailored according to where it is being implemented, or in the extent to which the premise for community interventions is locally generated. An approach inconsistent with the ecological approach would be one in which researchers recruit participants to test out concepts or hypotheses that are developed or selected solely by the researchers (Kingry-Westergaard & Kelly, 1990). This issue of collaboration and responsive engagement is highlighted as essential in a number of chapters within this text. Chapter 3 considers collaboration from the very outset of the research, reflecting on the development of tenders for research in cooperation with community stakeholders, while Chapter 5 explicitly focuses on working with these groups. On a practical level, Chapter 7 specifically examines how to prepare researcher teams for working in the community.

Community research conducted through an ecological lens also places great emphasis on the involvement of the community at all phases of the research process. Thus, the process is collaborative and participatory, and involves working with, rather than on, people (Nelson & Prilleltensky, 2010). Community members are not considered passive recipients in the research process. Kingry-Westergaard and Kelly (1990) suggest that collaborative relationships between the researcher and participants within the community setting give rise to an understanding of behaviour-in-context. The researcher–participant relationship becomes the source for the construction of meaning about whatever phenomenon is being studied. Persons and their systems are best understood when they are considered as part of a multi-level, multi-determined social context. This idea reflects a 'contextualist epistemology', where epistemology refers to the relationship between the researcher and what can be known (Guba & Lincoln, 2005). Knowledge and understanding is co-constructed by the researcher and participants in the community setting: the researcher becomes informed about phenomena in context, and concepts are revised as the collaborative relationship with participants evolves (Kingry-Westergaard & Kelly, 1990).

Application of ecological models in community research

In this section of the chapter we draw upon two examples to illustrate the application of the ecological model in community research. The first example describes a multi-level community mobilization plan developed to promote youth development and prevent violence (Hernandez-Cordero et al., 2011) and the second example describes the implementation of the Healthy Living Cambridge Kids programme (Chomitz et al., 2010; Healthy Children Taskforce, 2007).

The programme described by Hernandez-Cordero et al. (2011) was developed by the Columbia Centre for Youth Violence Prevention (CCYVP), part of the School of Public Health at Columbia University, in collaboration with the UNIDOS Inwood Coalition. The UNIDOS Inwood Coalition (UNIDOS) was founded in 2000 to promote community mobilization efforts to reduce the youth substance abuse problem in Inwood, a Manhattan neighbourhood characterized by a high population density (approximately 60,000 residents within an area of 1.5 square miles), a high proportion of Hispanic residents and a high proportion of female-headed households (Olson et al., 2006). Within one sub-area of the neighbourhood with approximately 25,000 residents, 44 per cent of families with children younger than eighteen years live below the poverty level.

This intervention adopted a multi-level approach to services coordination that utilizes and redirects current resources to serve young people. The plan was firmly embedded within an ecological framework and involved the development of individual-level, family-level, block-level, organizational-level and built environment-level activities. Partner groups, representing sectors such as youth, parents, schools/education, youth-serving organizations, business, law enforcement agencies, faith/civic/volunteering organizations, governmental agencies, substance abuse prevention/treatment agencies and public health agencies were given opportunities to contribute to the development and implementation of the plan.

Individual level activities were targeted at young people identified who had previously committed a minor offence and so were deemed to be at risk of delinquent behaviour, as well as at potential young leaders. Young people were connected with a resource, such as a group or individual counselling programme delivered by students taking a graduate programme in social work. A community intern position provided part-time work opportunities to those who had demonstrated leadership and were enrolled in an academic program. These interns brought to the plan a nuanced understanding of the community context and how to engage others in the plan.

Family-level interventions included family strengthening activities, such as the roll-out of a literacy programme to enhance parent–child bonding through dedicated reading time, and the Family to Family Program. This latter programme is a replication of the Family's Home Evening Enrichment program, developed to expand the social networks of families and children in impoverished communities in Harlem (Fullilove, Green & Fullilove, 2000). Block-level activities concentrated on specific areas in which delinquency and criminal activity were particularly high. The aim was to enhance protective factors within these 'hot spots' by strengthening block cohesiveness, encouraging collective youth supervision and increasing positive parenting. Organizational level activities involved exploring the feasibility of adapting existing programmes and services (such as after-school activities and access to computer centres) to expand the scope of their impact. At the built-environment level, focus was directed towards re-purposing public spaces usually feared by residents. Outdoor events were coordinated and messages were disseminated about the use of public spaces.

Aside from targeting multiple levels of context and mobilizing existing resources within the community, this intervention reflects the ecological approach in how the plan evolved and was implemented. University-based centres worked as partners in the process, not as conveners, and existing community-based organizations worked as catalysts to address multiple manifestations of youth violence and their determinants. Thus, different partners took on responsibility for leading specific work packages, but all work packages were complementary. The collective work of the CCYVP and the UNIDOS Coalition highlights the value of focused planning and mobilization of existing resources across multiple levels of context (Hernandez-Cordero et al., 2011).

Hernandez-Cordero et al. (2011) also highlight that the UNIDOS Coalition has chosen to use evidence-based practices in their community mobilization programme. However, the faithfulness with which various evidence-based programmes have been implemented has varied, depending upon factors such as cost, requirement for paid staff or volunteers, requirement for training and the applicability of the programme for specific populations and settings. Data have not yet been presented on the efficacy of the work in the community.

The second example describes a community-based intervention to promote healthy weight and fitness among children in Cambridge, Massachusetts (Chomitz et al., 2010). According to the authors, the study represents part of "an emerging grassroots childhood obesity prevention movement" (p. S46), in which the community mobilizes its resources to implement and evaluate a multi-pronged programme across multiple layers of the eco-system. At an individual and family level, policies were implemented to increase awareness of risk for obesity among children and their families and to provide skills and resources for addressing health risk factors. 'Fit Together' family event nights were organized and families of obese children were offered subsidized weight management counselling. At the school level, policies regarding physical activity and food service were implemented. For example, restrictions were placed upon certain items being sold in vending machines, and school menus were upgraded by including more fresh vegetables, seasonal produce from a local farm and less processed food. Schoolyard garden programmes were initiated to expand awareness of locally grown produce. Physical education (PE) in school was expanded to incorporate a range of non-traditional activities such as yoga and ballroom dance, and before- and after-school programming was expanded. At the community level, strategies were designed to provide policy support for healthy living choices, such as endorsement by the city council of the 5–2–1 guidelines (five portions of fruit/vegetables; less than two hours of screen time; one hour of physical activity per day). A poster campaign was initiated to raise community awareness of the many resources available in the city to promote healthy eating and active living, a youth sports commission was established and mini-grants were awarded to fifteen community-based organizations to promote the 5–2–1 guidelines.

The study adopted a community based participatory research (CBPR) approach in which community members were engaged in all aspects of the research process from design and implementation of the study to analysis, dissemination and consideration of the sustainability of the program. The study reflected a collaborative effort between the Healthy Children Task Force (multidisciplinary coalition of elected officials, educators, health care professionals, parents and researchers), the Institute for Community Health and the Cambridge Public Health Department. As noted in Chapter 1, CBPR is a critical approach in effective research with communities.

The efficacy of the intervention has been evaluated by means of pre- and post-test measurement of children's fitness and body mass index (BMI), both measured by PE teachers and school nurses. Modest improvements in obesity and fitness were observed among children from baseline to follow-up (three-year period). The authors suggest that the results speak to the importance of long-term commitment of community resources and innovation necessary for addressing the problem of childhood obesity. While children in all racial/ethnic and income groups demonstrated improvements in weight status, Hispanic and Black children continued to show elevated rates of obesity, suggesting that intervention approaches that specifically target each community may be needed. The evaluation was limited in that there was no control group; thus the changes in BMI and fitness cannot be solely attributed to the intervention, but could be due to a more general secular shift caused by the increased attention directed at the problem of childhood obesity. Finally, it is not possible to identify which elements of the intervention contributed to the changes in BMI or fitness.

We consider the challenges inherent to conducting community research in full in the final section of this chapter. It is, however, noteworthy that the ecological model alone may be limited as a research theory because it fails to account for differential levels of power that individuals may have which might shape how they interact with their environment (Nelson & Prilleltensky, 2010). This issue of power has been addressed by empowerment theories, which will be considered next.

Empowerment approaches to community research

Given the importance of respect for individuals and their contexts that ecological approaches to research embody, empowerment theories can be seen as naturally complementary approaches. Theories of empowerment have their roots in the work by Brazilian humanitarian Freire (2000), who conceived of empowerment as a means of changing the life course of oppressed people via education. Since then, many theories of empowerment have been put forth (Cattaneo & Chapman, 2010; Chinman & Linney, 1998; Foster-Fishman et al., 1998; Hur, 2006; Rappaport, 1987; Speer, Jackson & Peterson, 2001; Zimmerman, 1995), and researchers across disciplines have refined both the definition of empowerment and the processes by which empowerment occurs (e.g. Peterson, 2014). Although empowerment as a concept is cited as an important factor in multiple research disciplines, a definitive definition of empowerment remains elusive (Hur, 2006). Yet, for those interested in community change and research, empowerment remains both a value (Rappaport, 1987), a goal (Zimmerman, 1995) and a process by which positive community change is achieved (Cattaneo & Chapman, 2010). Furthermore, theories of empowerment shape the kinds of research conducted in community settings and have given way to new approaches to research such as CBPR, a research method illustrated above that emphasizes community stakeholders as equal partners to academics, policy-makers and funders in community research efforts. In the following sections of this chapter we explore the nature and definition of empowerment in the context of community research. We then highlight theories of empowerment and examples of community research informed by these theories.

Empowerment defined

At its essence, empowerment is the base process by which people's lives and circumstances are improved (Cattaneo & Chapman, 2010). This process involves the ways in which individuals and communities gain access to knowledge and resources that allow for greater control and choice over future outcomes (Rappaport, 1984; Zimmerman, 2000). These resources may encompass many things at many ecological levels, dependent on goal and circumstance. Some resources that might contribute to the process of empowerment may be monetary, intellectual or political in nature. Most resources associated with empowerment are explicitly linked to acquiring skills, knowledge or clout in order to achieve specified goals. Modern definitions of empowerment suggest that empowerment is a dynamic process that can be conceptualized in terms of ecological principles, as empowerment is multi-dimensional and occurs at both the individual and community level (Hur, 2006). It is also influenced by macro-level systems such as political, cultural and economic contexts (Hur, 2006).

Rappaport proposes a simple and all-encompassing definition of empowerment. According to Rappaport (1984, p. 3), empowerment is the "mechanism by which people, organizations and communities gain mastery over their lives". Expanding on this definition is the notion that empowerment is a process, not a destination (Cargo, et al., 2003), indicating that the steps taken toward empowerment are valuable and empowering in and of themselves. In support of this notion, Rappaport (1987) suggests that individuals gain power via initiatives that emphasize active collaborative participation, an acknowledgement of differences and an emphasis on strengths.

An appreciation and respect for individual and cultural differences is paramount to successful empowerment processes, as factors that lead to empowerment are determined by characteristics of the individual as well as their environment (Zimmerman, 2000). Furthermore, empowerment is an interactional process (Zimmerman, 2000). Since empowerment processes reflect a unique experience and emphasize strengths and collaboration, research initiatives that emphasize empowerment may be uniquely suited for those who may be disadvantaged or feel disenfranchised. As an example, programmes aimed at serving youth often emphasize activities that enhance identity development, bonding and social control (Chinman & Linney, 1998). Moreover, these kinds of approaches to youth empowerment such as community participation have been shown to have protective effects on adolescent health and wellbeing (Cargo, et al., 2003).

Keeping the notions of empowerment in mind, in order for community participation in research to be meaningful to those involved, it needs to be genuine, promoting the voice of those who may have historically been excluded from community decision making and policy development (Lasker & McGuidry, 2009). Mere involvement in a given research programme or initiative is not sufficient to assure meaningful engagement among participating partners, however. In a study of factors that contribute to community involvement, Speer, Jackson and Peterson (2001) found that those who reported more cohesion with other community members were more likely to report higher levels of empowerment despite similar levels of community involvement. These findings indicate that individuals need to feel a part of those research programmes aimed at empowerment.

As illustrated above, empowerment does not happen in a vacuum. It is the process of working with others that builds resources and competencies. To create an environment where people feel welcomed and comfortable, it is necessary to have elements of social cohesion (Speer et al., 2001). Factors that contribute to cohesion are trust, connectedness and civic engagement (Speer et al., 2001). Those who conduct research informed by empowerment theory take these complex interactions into account, so that ideally community members are an integral and valued part of the planning and implementation processes of community initiatives. In the following section, we consider empowerment process models and highlight two community projects as examples of research informed by empowerment theory.

The research process conducted through an empowerment lens

Because empowerment theory can seem vague, it is important to have a good working model of how empowerment takes place. For this reason, recent models of empowerment attempt to further refine the empowerment process. Cattaneo and Chapman (2010) conceive of empowerment as goal directed and action oriented. According to this model, empowerment is conceptualized as a cyclical process where individual self-efficacy, knowledge and competence all work together within a social context and individuals define their goals, carry out plans to achieve these goals and reflect upon the impact of their actions (Cattaneo & Chapman, 2010). Furthermore, Hur (2006) extensively reviewed components of empowerment to identify common processes across disciplines. This work concluded that empowerment is experienced at both the individual and community levels and several components at each of these levels were identified. At the individual level, these factors include *meaning, competence, self-determination* and *impact*. At the community level, these factors include *belonging, community involvement, organizational control* and *community building*. Although research informed by empowerment would ideally target both individual and community empowerment, the following examples will be used as a way to highlight each of these components of the theory.

Individual empowerment in community research

To illustrate how each of the components of Hur's individual empowerment can be used to inform community research, we will consider a community research project that utilized a form of CBPR known as photovoice to investigate homelessness in Auckland, New Zealand.

Photovoice is a method of CBPR that embraces the tenets of empowerment (Wallerstein & Bernstein, 1988; Wang & Burris, 1994, 1997), as CBPR methodologies can be utilized to address social and environmental inequities (Castledon, Mulrenan & Godlewska, 2012). Like all forms of CBPR, photovoice entails a partnership between researchers and community members in an effort to understand a community challenge or phenomenon. Although many individuals may share views, backgrounds and life events, each person experiences the world around them in their own unique way. Photovoice is a community research method that gives people an opportunity to share their lived experiences through photos and narrative. In this way, it allows people who may not usually be heard to make their views and stories known (Winchester, 2000). Often, decisions on how to help a given disadvantaged group such as children, the poor and those diagnosed with mental illness are made without direct input from these individuals. Photovoice can be used as a needs assessment tool, as it allows individual experiences to be documented and analysed. It can also be an effective way to highlight inequities, so that community needs can be addressed.

Homelessness is an issue facing many large metropolitan areas (Glasser, 1994). Much of the research on homelessness focuses on the plight of homeless men (Bukowski & Buetow, 2010). However, as economic climates change, women and children are increasingly affected by homelessness, and recent community research reflects these changes. The life circumstances and risks of homeless women may be different from those of homeless men (Glasser, 1994). In order to address these issues, Bukowski and Buetow (2010) conducted a photovoice study of homeless women in Auckland, NZ. This study provided a small sample of homeless women in Auckland with cameras, so that they could photographically document their experiences of life on the streets. It also provided an opportunity for participants to discuss the meaning of what was depicted in the photographs. Along with providing opportunities for participants to document and discuss their experiences, researchers also gathered demographic and health information relevant to the study. Participants took photographs of various subjects, including makeshift beds and food preparation. Some of the themes of this study included the dangers associated with homelessness, aspects of the social support within the homeless community and feelings about social and health care services (Bukowski & Buetow, 2010). One of the key findings of the study was that participants were able to identify leaders within their own community who might be able to liaise with homelessness programmes in an effort to improve services for homeless women in Auckland.

This research is an example of an effort to create opportunities for individual empowerment across all the four factors identified by Hur (2006) – meaning, competence, self-determination and impact. Participants in this study were arguably amongst the most disenfranchised in any community population, yet taking part in the photovoice project may have added meaning to their daily acts of survival, as researchers respected participant individuality and voice. Through these endeavours, members of the community were free to choose to be a part of the study and express themselves through photography the way they saw fit. This is a simple example of *self-determination*. The photographs taken by participants in the programme served as a means for discussion and informed efforts to improve services. These efforts proved that participants were valued and had the necessary *competence* to make their stories known. Therefore, their work did not just represent a futile exercise but a very *meaningful* contribution to community change efforts. Given future directions were based in part by participant input, those who participated had real *impact* on their circumstances and future.

Community empowerment in community research

To illustrate how each of the components of Hur's community empowerment theory – *belonging, community involvement, organizational control* and *community building* – can be used to inform community research, we will consider a grassroots community research project aimed at improving school readiness for disadvantaged children in Dublin, Ireland.

Social disadvantage is associated with increased risk across a number of domains (Luthar, 1999). The intergenerational transmission of socioeconomic inequalities in children's health and cognitive, behavioural and emotional development emerge early, and can persist through life (Luthar, 1999; Masten, Best & Garmezy, 1990). The Preparing for Life Programme (PFL) was created to address these issues. PFL is a mentor-based home visiting programme. The goal of PFL is to intervene during pregnancy and work with families until children start school to improve levels of school readiness across a number of domains (Doyle, 2012). This intervention includes one-on-one mentoring with a professional mentor, as well as group parenting training and opportunities for parents to socialize. PFL was a bottom-up initiative, which was five years in development. Over 20 local agencies and community organizations worked collaboratively to develop this programme. The research evaluation component was designed in conjunction with the programme itself. A high level of engagement from respected and well-established community agencies set the stage for strong support and community 'buy in' throughout the life of PFL. The planning and steering committees that guide this programme included individuals from a wide range of backgrounds and expertise, including government officials, educators, funders, health care professionals, academics and parents from the community.

Community members played a vital role in developing PFL and continue to shape the direction of the programme. In the context of the PFL programme, community member roles are varied. They are trusted community partners, as community members are involved with PFL's parent organization, Northside Partnership, an organization that aims to counter disadvantage and promote equality and social and economic inclusion within the community. They are community experts. Members of the community sit on the steering committee and have been involved in programme planning and governance since its inception. They are programme experts. As part of the PFL evaluation, focus groups are held regularly with participants to gain valuable feedback regarding programme successes and challenges. PFL participants are the advocates for the programme, as they regularly meet with government officials and funding bodies on behalf of the programme.

Each of Hur's (2006) community level elements of empowerment is evidenced in the development and implementation of the PFL programme and evaluation. *Community involvement* is reflected in the development and governance of PFL. Community members from various backgrounds work collaboratively to shape and inform the programme. This gives the community some margin of *organizational control* of the programme. The community has input in the current and future directions of the programme. The programme is designed to promote a sense of *belonging* within the community by creating opportunities for community members to learn and socialize. Both belonging and involvement help *build a stronger community*, one where citizens feel they are a part of something beyond kinship with their immediate family.

Challenges of ecological and empowerment models

As illustrated by the examples provided in this chapter, the value of ecological and empowerment approaches for understanding individuals and their environments is widely accepted. However, the complexity inherent in these models brings many challenges for those involved in community research. The outcomes associated with community intervention must be clearly conceived, and outcomes appropriate for each level of multi-level interventions should be defined and measured separately. Unintended outcomes should also be considered, and anticipatory and surveillance processes are important for monitoring ripple effects that may occur (Trickett & Schensul, 2009). The challenges of communicating unexpected findings is considered in detail in Chapter 9 of this text, including reflecting on the potential impact of these messages on community stakeholders and offering strategies to maintain trust in these situations. Further, the collaboration and relationships among participating groups and organizations need to be considered, as these reflect an important element of the process. Different forms of data and data from different sources may need to be triangulated in order to gain a comprehensive understanding of what is going on. Trickett and Schensul (2009) document further challenges inherent in aligning an ecologically based programme with a rigorous evaluation process. Specifically, they note that activities at other levels of community systems may interact in unpredicted, unmeasured and uncontrollable ways, thus representing a threat to the validity of a quasi-experiment or randomized controlled design.

Conclusion

Conventional approaches to community research may not be successful, as they may fail to take those they wish to serve into account. This is a common theme throughout this text, with multiple chapters considering the need to be responsive to the range of stakeholders in community-based research, and practical strategies for maximising buy-in and engagement considered in key areas. Research that is informed by ecological and empowerment theories recognizes that in order to conduct sound community research, it is necessary for community members to be full partners in research endeavours. Although the process of collaboration between researchers and community members may be challenging, the examples included in this chapter illustrate that it is possible for people from diverse backgrounds to work collaboratively. When community members are engaged in the planning, implementation and evaluation processes of community research, sustainable community change is possible.

References

Bronfenbrenner, U. (1979) *The ecology of human development: Experiments in nature and design*. Cambridge, MA: Harvard University Press.

Bronfenbrenner, U. (1993) 'The ecology of cognitive development: Research models and fugitive findings', in Wonziak, R. & Fischer, K. (eds) *Development in contexts: Acting and thinking in specific environments*. Hillsdale, NJ: Erlbaum, pp. 3–44.

Bronfenbrenner, U. (2005) *Making human beings human: Bioecological perspectives on human development*. Thousand Oaks, CA: SAGE.

Bronfenbrenner, U. & Morris, P.A. (2006) 'The bioecological model of human development', in Damon, W. (series ed) & Lerner, R.M. (vol. ed) *Handbook of child psychology: Vol. 1. Theoretical models of human development*. 6th edn. New York, NY: Wiley, pp. 793–828.

Bukowski, K. & Buetow, S. (2011) 'Making the invisible visible: A photovoice exploration of homeless women's health and lives in central Auckland', *Social Science & Medicine*, 72, pp. 739–746.

Cargo, M. *et al.* (2003) 'Empowerment as fostering positive youth development and citizenship', *American Journal of Health Behaviour*, 27, pp. S66–S79.

Castleden, H., Mulrennan, M. & Godlewska, A. (2012) 'Community-based participatory research involving Indigeneous peoples in Canadian geography: Progress? An editorial introduction', *Canadian Geographer*, 56, pp. 155–159.

Cattaneo, L.B. & Chapman, A.R. (2010) 'The process of empowerment: A model for use in research and practice', *American Psychologist*, 65, pp. 646–659.

Chinman, M.J. & Linney, J.A. (1998) 'Toward a model of adolescent empowerment: Theoretical and empirical evidence', *The Journal of Primary Prevention*, 18, pp. 393–413.

Chomitz, V.R. *et al.* (2010) 'Healthy Living Cambridge Kids: A community-based participatory effort to promote healthy weight and fitness', *Obesity*, 18 (Supplement 1), pp. S43–S53.

Dallos, R. & Draper, R. (2010) *An introduction to family therapy: Systemic theory and practice*. 3rd edn. Berkshire, England: McGraw Hill/Open University Press.

Doyle, O. (2012) 'Breaking the Cycle of Deprivation: An Experimental Evaluation of an Early Childhood Intervention', Presentation to the Statistical & Social Inquiry Society of Ireland, Royal Irish Academy. April.

Foster-Fishman, P.G. *et al.* (1998) 'Empirical support for the critical assumptions of empowerment theory', *American Journal of Community Psychology*, 26, pp. 507–536.

Freire, P. (2000) *Pedagogy of the oppressed*. New York, NY: Continuum. (Original work published 1970).

Fullilove, R.E., Green, L. & Fullilove, M.T. (2000) 'The family to family program: A structural intervention with implications for the prevention of HIV/AIDS and other community epidemics', *AIDS*, 14, pp. S63–S67.

Glasser, I. (1994) *Homelessness in global perspective*. New York, NY: MacMillan.

Guba, E.G. & Lincoln, Y.S. (2005) 'Paradigmatic controversies, contradictions, and emerging confluences, in Denzin, N.K. & Lincoln, Y.S. (eds) *The Sage handbook of qualitative research*. 3rd edn. Thousand Oaks, CA: SAGE, pp. 191–215.

Healthy Children Taskforce (2007) Healthy Living Cambridge Kids. Cambridge, Massachusetts. Available from www.icommunityhealth.org/documents/publications/HealthyLivingCambridgeKids.pdf (Accessed on 6 July 2012).

Hernandez-Cordero, L.J. *et al.* (2011) 'Fresh start: A multilevel community mobilization plan to promote youth development and prevent violence', *American Journal of Community Psychology*, 48, pp. 43–55.

Hur, M.H. (2006) 'Empowerment in terms of theoretical perspectives: Exploring a typology of the process and components across disciplines', *Journal of Community Psychology*, 34, pp. 523–540.

Kelly, J.G. (1966) 'Ecological constraints on mental health', *American Psychologist*, 21, pp. 535–539.

Kelly, J.G. (1968) 'Toward an ecological concept of preventive interventions', in Carter, J. (ed) *Research contributions from psychology to community mental health*. New York, NY: Behavioural Publications, pp. 75–99.

Kelly, J.G. (1971) 'Qualities for the community psychologist', *American Psychologist*, 26, pp. 897–903.

Kelly, J.G. (2006) *Becoming ecological: An expedition into community psychology*. Oxford: Oxford University Press.

Kelly, J.G. *et al.* (2000) 'Understanding and changing social systems. An ecological view', in Rappaport, J. & Seidman, E. (eds) *Handbook of community psychology*. New York: Kluwer Academic/Plenum Publishers, pp. 133–159.

Kingry-Westergaard, C. & Kelly, J.G. (1990) 'A contextualist epistemology for ecological research', in Tolan, P. *et al.* (eds) *Research community psychology: Issues for theory and methods*. Washington DC: American Psychological Association, pp. 23–31.

Klein, D.M. & White, J.M. (1996) *Family theories: An introduction*. Thousand Oaks, CA: SAGE.

Lasker, R.D. & McGuidry, A. (2009) *Engaging the community in decision making: Case studies tracking participation, voice and influence*. Jefferson, NC: McFarland & Co. Inc. Publishers.

Luthar, S.S. (1999) *Poverty and children's adjustment*. Thousand Oaks, CA: SAGE.

Masten, A.S., Best, K.M. & Garmezy, N. (1990) 'Resilience and development: Contributions from the study of children who overcome adversity', *Development and Psychopathology*, 2, pp. 425–444.

Nelson, G. & Prilleltensky, I. (2010) *Community psychology: In pursuit of liberation and well-being*. 2nd edn. New York, NY: Palgrave Macmillan.

Olson, E. *et al.* (2006). 'Take Care Inwood and Washington Heights', *NYC community health profiles*. 2nd edn. Available from www1.nyc.gov/assets/doh/downloads/pdf/data/2006chp-301.pdf (Accessed 15 May 2017).

Peirson, L.J. *et al.* (2011) 'An ecological process model of systems change', *American Journal of Community Psychology*, 47, pp. 301–321.

Peterson, N.A. (2014) 'Empowerment theory: Clarifying the nature of higher-order multidimensional constructs', *American Journal of Community Psychology*, 53, pp. 96–108.

Prilleltensky, I. & Nelson, G. (2009) 'Community psychology. Advancing social justice', in Fox, D., Prilleltensky, I. & Austin, S. (eds) *Critical psychology: An introduction*. 2nd edn. London: SAGE, pp. 126–143.

Rappaport, J. (1981) 'In praise of paradox: A social policy of empowerment over prevention', *American Journal of Community Psychology*, 9, pp. 1–25.

Rappaport, J. (1984) 'Studies in empowerment: Introduction to the issues,' in Rappaport, J., Swift, C. and Hess, R. (eds) *Studies in empowerment: Steps toward understanding and action*. New York, NY: The Haworth Press, pp. 1–7.

Rappaport, J. (1987) 'Terms of empowerment/exemplars of prevention: Toward a theory for community psychology', *American Journal of Community Psychology*, 15, pp. 121–148.

Speer, P.W., Jackson, C.B. & Peterson, N.A. (2001) 'The relationship between social cohesion and empowerment: Support and new implications for theory', *Health Education & Behavior*, 28, pp. 716–732.

Trickett, E.J. (1986) 'Consultation as a preventive intervention: Comments on ecologically based case studies', *Prevention in Human Services*, 4, pp. 187–204.

Trickett, E.J. (1996) 'A future for community psychology: The contexts of diversity and the diversity of contexts', *American Journal of Community Psychology*, 24, pp. 209–234.

Trickett, E.J. (2009) 'Multilevel community-based culturally situated interventions and community impact: An ecological perspective', *American Journal of Community Psychology*, 43, pp. 257–266.

Trickett, E.J., Kelly, J.G. & Todd, D.M. (1972) 'The social environment of the high school: Guidelines for individual change and organizational redevelopment', in Golann, S.E. & Eisdorfer, C. (eds) *Handbook of community mental health*. New York, NY: Appleton-Century-Crofts, pp. 331–406.

Trickett, E.J., Kelly, J.G. & Vincent, T.A. (1985) 'The spirit of ecological inquiry in community research', in Susskind, E.C. & Klein, D.C. (eds) *Community research*. New York, NY: Praeger, pp. 283–333.

Trickett, E.J. & Schensul, J.J. (2009) 'Summary comments: Multi-level community based culturally situated interventions', *American Journal of Community Psychology*, 43, pp. 377–381.

Tudge, J.R.H. *et al.* (2009) 'Uses and misuses of Bronfenbrenner's bioecological theory of human development', *Journal of Family Theory & Review*, 1, pp. 198–210.

Tudge, J.R.H. *et al.* (2016) 'Still misused after all these years? A re-evaluation of the uses of Bronfenbrenner's bioecological theory of human development', *Journal of Family Theory and Review*, 8, pp. 425–445.

Wallerstein, N. & Bernstein, E. (1988) 'Empowerment education: Freire's ideas adapted to health education', *Health Education & Behaviour*, 15, pp. 379–394.

Wang, C. & Burris, M.A. (1994) 'Empowerment through photo novella', *Health Education Quarterly*, 21, pp. 171–186.

Wang, C. & Burris, M.A. (1997) 'Photovoice: Concept, methodology, and use for participatory needs assessment', *Health Education & Behaviour*, 24, pp. 369–387.

WangC. *et al.* (1998) 'Photovoice as a participatory health promotion strategy', *Health Promotion International*, 13, pp. 75–87.

Winchester, H. (2000) 'Qualitative research and its place in human geography', in Hay, I. (ed) *Qualitative research methods in human geography*. Melbourne: Oxford University Press.

Winegar, L.T. (1997) 'Developmental research and comparative perspectives: Applications to developmental science', in Tudge, J., Shanahan, M.J. & Valsiner, J. (eds) *Comparisons in human development: Understanding time and context*. Cambridge: Cambridge University Press, pp. 13–33.

Zimmerman, M.A. (1995) 'Psychological empowerment: Issues and illustrations', *American Journal of Community Psychology*, 23, pp. 581–599.

Zimmerman, M.A. (2000) 'Empowerment theory: Psychological, organizational, and community levels of analysis', in Rappaport, J. & Seidman, E. (eds) *Handbook of community psychology*. New York, NY: Kluwer Academic/Plenum, pp. 43–63.

3 Commissioning, procuring and contracting evaluations and research

Marian Quinn, Catherine Comiskey and Gail Birkbeck

Introduction

Whilst both the voluntary and statutory sectors have a history of reliance on external supports to evaluate services, programmes and processes, the context of these relationships has significantly changed in recent years for a number of reasons, including a deepened understanding of the need for accountability, added value and appropriate use of funding. This has raised issues relating to ownership of data, approval mechanisms for publishing reports and the appropriate timing and fora in which to interpret and share findings.

Alongside these discussions, some child, family and community services in Ireland have received considerable investment to support evaluations, many including more rigorous, scientific methods than would previously have been utilized. For example, chapters in this book draw on examples of randomized controlled trials conducted in service settings following such investment. This has brought challenges as well as opportunities, particularly in relation to issues such as information feedback loops, keeping stakeholders on board whilst avoiding any impact on programme outcomes, the potential for research burden and the approach to and timing of dissemination so that it maximizes learning without undermining the rigour of the research. Whilst these issues will be addressed more comprehensively in other chapters in this book, they are relevant to the procurement process, as they point to the need for consideration of legal ownership and contractual clarity of the data and outputs from research.

This chapter has been written with the objective of providing guidance for those wishing to either commission research and evaluation or respond to such invitations and as such is instructional and directive in nature. Whilst the participation of and engagement with the community is referenced, and indeed encouraged in the context of community based research, the nature of procurement, the contractual relationships resulting from this process and the sometimes significant funding involved, means that there is generally limited space for partners other than the commissioner and the researcher to directly engage in this phase.

The chapter draws on the experience of a range of settings, processes and evaluation models, as well as the legislative and regulatory context, bringing together some key principles and good practice frameworks. It should be noted that whilst the chapter takes a broadly chronological approach to the various steps involved in commissioning and contracting research, in reality it is likely that these phases will merge and be revisited and that there will be some movement between them as clarity is gained.

For the purposes of this chapter, the following terms will be used:

- 'The commissioner' or 'commissioning agent' refers to the organization seeking to recruit external support with research or evaluation processes. This may be a public sector body, a voluntary organization or a community organization.
- 'Researcher' refers to the individual or organization responding to an invitation to undertake research or evaluation on behalf of the commissioner. This may be an academic institution, a commercial organization, a public sector body or an individual.
- 'Request for Tender' refers to the formal invitation to researchers to submit a proposal for the services required.

Underpinning principles

In the past, commissioning agents have tended to be weak in relation to monitoring, accountability and ownership of data resulting from research they have supported. Indeed, commissioners may be unaware of the extent of the data they hold or have access to, the possible uses of these data and the knowledge that can be gained from them. One such example is in substance misuse services, where organizations often obtain data from complex families with multiple needs, including information about the children of parents who use drugs and how parental drug use has changed over time (Meir, Donmall & McElduff, 2004; Comiskey, 2013; Comiskey & Snel, 2016). These data might not be the primary focus of the organization, but they offer a wealth of opportunities for understanding the needs of the families of service users.

The academic community has tended to have ownership of research and evaluation findings, possibly due to European taxation systems, which offer preferential allowances to these types of contracts (Office of the Revenue Commissioners, n.d.). Ownership of course generally determines when and what gets published, although of course the reverse is also true, where evaluations have been undertaken and the commissioning agent, possibly due to the conclusions drawn from the research, has failed to utilize the findings or publicize them in any meaningful way. Neither of these situations makes for a healthy, vibrant dialogue based on learning, insights and evidence which could inform future policy and practice.

It has been suggested that the key to an effective, workable and appropriate use of data is the relationship between the commissioner and the researcher, and the need for a respectful and honest rapport is critical. An inequity of power or lack of clarity regarding ownership and expectations will be problematic if contentious issues arise, which they almost inevitably will. The procurement process and subsequent contractual obligations can support or mitigate against such a relationship. For example, Chapter 10 refers to the management of negative evaluation findings, and illustrates the centrality of the partnership approach undertaken by the research team and the commissioning agent.

In addition, organizations seeking to commission independent community based research, and perhaps move towards more evidence informed approaches, should consider and recognize the tensions that are inherent in this:

> there is a great tension between working in a community development fashion while also designing, implementing and evaluating, to a very high level, a set of manualised programmes.
>
> (Canavan et al., 2014, p. 48)

Taking an evidence informed approach, often supported by access to experts and existing research, necessarily reduces the role of the community. Giving this some consideration, particularly in relation to appropriate and respectful mechanisms through which service users can inform the work, may minimize tensions later in the research process.

The following outlines the key principles found to be central to developing and maintaining effective relationships between the researcher and the commissioner:

- Allowing time for the procurement process is a sound investment of resources. It can be a very lengthy one, but this is one of the most important decisions a commissioner will make, so commit the time to ensure there is a good fit between the expectations and needs of the commissioner and the expertise, skills and working methods of the researcher. Approaching the procurement like a recruitment process maximizes the types of checks which can inform decisions. For example, the commissioning agent can take up references and hold interviews whilst the researcher may find out about the organization, what their ethos is, how they work and what exactly they are looking for. Establishing this information will contribute to a positive partnership.
- Building in monitoring and review opportunities from the outset can be a more effective and proactive step than having to respond later in the process if a problem arises.
- Obtaining a balance between clarity and flexibility will support effective communication. Too much of the former can be stifling and restrictive, whilst an over emphasis on the latter can be confusing. There is a middle ground to be achieved.
- It can be very helpful if commissioners are explicit about their key requirements, areas for compromise and those where this is not possible. For example, give consideration to the ownership and publication of data.

- Considering the role of various partners (such as community representatives, service users or technical experts) and how they might inform the evaluation process can bring valuable and rich insights. Agree how they will be involved at the outset or ensure space to later reflect on how they might be involved.
- Recognize that the process will be easier and more productive if the parties involved have a well-functioning relationship. There needs to be a sense of trust that if there is a problem, the commissioning agent and the researchers will be able to talk it through and resolve it.

Building on these general principles, Table 3.1 outlines some specific issues that the commissioning agent and the researcher may need to consider.

Gaining clarity regarding the above will inform the content of both the Request for Tender (RFT) document, which the commissioner circulates, and the contract that will ultimately be signed by both the commissioner and the researcher.

Procurement procedures

The basic principle underpinning effective and appropriate procurement is that it allows for and facilitates an open, competitive process and that selection is undertaken in an objective and non-discriminatory way. In Ireland, both public sector bodies and organizations that receive 50% or more funding from the state are required to adhere to both the Irish and European regulations (https://ec.europa.eu/growth/single-market/public-procurement_en), whilst the World Trade Organization (WTO) has well established procedures for the international procurement of services using government funding (WTO, 2014). Whilst other organizations such as those privately funded or operating for commercial purposes have no obligation to adhere to these principles, the authors suggest that in the interests of good practice and transparency, the guidelines set out below be considered by all.

The appropriate mechanism by which a procurement contract is circulated and ultimately awarded is informed by the budget allocated to the piece of work to be commissioned. The greater the budget, the more open and transparent the process should be. The thresholds for these levels of procurement may change, and are available from the relevant websites (see Table 3.2). At the time of print, they are as follows for research and development contracts:

- Under €1,000: The guidelines state that a "number sufficient to allow for competition" should be invited to tender. Generally, three verbal quotes from competitive suppliers are regarded as appropriate. The commissioner can target individuals and/or organizations to provide a quote.
- €1,000 to €25,000: The same principles as above apply, but at this value quotes should be provided in writing. Again, three submissions are acceptable, at a minimum.

Table 3.1 Issues for consideration by commissioners and researchers

For the commissioner	• Do you want to own all the data? If so, what consent will be required from participants? Where and how will you hold the data? How will you ensure it remains confidential? • What are your obligations under national/regional data protection legislation, for example the Data Protection Acts 1998 and 2003? • If you are commissioning an academic institution to undertake work, they will be required to receive ethical approval from their institution. Does their ethical approval fit with your expectations? • If you commission an independent researcher or company, what assurances will you need regarding the ethics of their approach, methodology, storing of data, etc. in the absence of an institutional ethics review process? • How will you respond if the research identifies negative findings, for example an evaluation that indicates that you are not achieving your stated objectives? How will you manage this? Who will you share this with? • What level of control do you need/want in relation to disseminating the findings from the research? • Is there other research going on in the area under your responsibility which needs to be considered? Do you need to agree a process by which time frames for data collection, review and publication are finalized? Who gets to decide these?
For the researcher	• Do you need to hold the data gathered as part of the research? Can you share any of it for further research? If so, with whom, and what consent is needed? • What does your local ethical approval process require of you? Does this fit with your contractual obligations to the commissioner? • How flexible can you be in relation to the timelines for data collection, analysis, interim reports and publication? If something happens in the community which impacts on your work, will you be in a position to respond, adapt, and amend? • What do you need in terms of opportunity to publish findings and utilize the learning in your work? Do you anticipate using the data for teaching or other learning exchanges? • If there are logistical difficulties with the fieldwork (e.g. lower than anticipated participation rates) do you know who to talk to about this? Are you confident of the commissioner's support?

Table 3.2 Some Useful Links

– www.activelink.ie – Used to advertise grants for research and evaluation
– www.dataprotection.ie – Guidance on data protection legislation
– www.etender.gov.ie – Irish website for public sector bodies advertising tenders
– http:://SIMAP.eu.int – Website for public sector bodies advertising tenders that reach European thresholds
– http://www.hrb.ie/ – Health Research Board (HRB)
– www.patentsopffice.ie – Irish Patents Office
– http://www.research.ie/ – Irish Research Council (IRC)
– http://www.nda.ie/ – National Disability Authority (NDA)
– http://www.ncse.ie/ – National Council for Special Education (NCSE)
– http://strobe-statement.org/index.php?id=available-checklists – Checklist for reporting observational studies

- €25,000 to €200,000: All contracts over €25,000 should be advertised on www.etenders.gov.ie, although it is also acceptable to supplement this by inviting individuals and/or organizations to make a submission.
- Over €200,000: Contracts that exceed this limit must adhere to the European Procurement Regulations, which require advertising the contract on the information system for European public procurement http://simap.ted.europa.eu/. There are also regulations regarding timelines for applications, which are available on the website.

Whichever process is applicable to the relevant jurisdiction, there are core principles and guidelines which apply and should be in place before an RFT can be issued or advertised. Timelines for submission of the procurement documentation should be clearly stated in the invitation, and should reflect the complexity and breadth of the work being contracted. The document should also state the time frame in which submissions will be reviewed and when applicants will be notified of a decision. It is important to note that late or incomplete submissions should not be accepted. With regard to the process of decision making, independent observation of or participation in the scoring process may be appropriate, especially if specific expertise is required to competently review submissions. Upon completion of the review process, score sheets should be signed and filed appropriately. Finally, mechanisms to provide feedback to unsuccessful applicants should be considered and agreed in advance of advertising the tender.

Developing, circulating and advertising an RFT

The key issue for any commissioning agent to consider when developing an RFT document is: How flexible would the commissioning agent like to be, or how flexible can they be? There is a balance to be struck between securing the desired work product (given the financial outlay) and being open to other ideas and perspectives that the researcher may bring to the process. The research team will have extensive expertise, so the commissioner will want to ensure opportunities are maximized to draw on this. In addition, the research team may engage more effectively if they have some ownership of the process, or if it fits with their own strengths, ethos and interests. Being clear in the RFT that there are areas that can be shaped by the research team and stating what these are will be very helpful for those responding.

An obvious but not necessarily simple first step in developing an RFT is to consider what programme of work or service is to be evaluated. The existence of a logic model underpinning any service or programme (see Murphy, Murphy & Smith 2011 for a description of this process) can provide the framework for the document. A logic model is a widely used process for planning a service or programme that meets identified needs (Murphy et al., 2011), and is based on a process that clarifies the identified needs being addressed by the programme of work, the research relating to effective interventions with regard to these needs and the actions to be undertaken to meet these needs. Ideally a logic model will be informed by local and national data; best practice and research regarding effective interventions; and local insights in terms of priority needs, available resources and the specific context. Therefore, a community consultation process should be undertaken alongside desk research. Developing a logic model is a useful process for any organization to undertake in relation to services and programmes, irrespective of independent evaluations. It is, however, particularly important if the aim is to assess the extent to which stated outcomes are being achieved.

In considering the key questions to focus on, the evaluation might therefore consider whether the identified needs have been met through the agreed actions, and possibly the relevance and usefulness of the literature underpinning the logic model (McCawley, 2001). It may also give attention to process elements of the service, or the 'how' of the work. For example, if inter-agency collaboration has been improved, what processes enabled this? What is the learning from the methods used to engage parents? Or how did the organization facilitate community participation?

In addition to identifying the key research questions to be answered, there are other areas to be considered before embarking on recruiting a researcher, which are presented in Table 3.3.

There are other questions that will need to be considered, but which may be best thought through with the evaluation team. The parties might consider how they can ensure the meaningful participation of the research's key target groups and what research methods would be most appropriate for the target group, given what is known about them. A particular challenge might be avoiding research fatigue among key stakeholders (Soukeriah & Tannock, 2013). Finally, it can be helpful to consider what feedback loops will sustain involvement and enthusiasm amongst stakeholders, including how to inform key groups about lessons learned and how to involve them in the interpretation of data.

With or without a logic model, the ideal starting point is to establish a small working group to draw up the tender document. Ideally, this group

Table 3.3 Key decisions and influencers

- Why does the commissioner require an evaluation? Is it because we really want to learn about whether we are impacting on identified needs? Is it because our funding requires it? Or because we might get extra funding if the evaluation is positive?
- How much money is available to the commissioner? What can we afford?
- What are the key timelines? Is there a specific date by which we need the report? How flexible are we?
- Are there histories, relationships or sensitivities the commissioner needs to be cognisant of? For example, is there research overload in this community already? Have some of the stakeholders had negative experiences of evaluations in the past? If so, how can we reassure them about this process?

should include someone with research expertise, someone with a working knowledge of the service or programme to be evaluated and someone who knows the community and its history well. Additionally, the experience of someone who has commissioned research elsewhere could be helpful to this working group, even if they only review its draft documents. The working group should have clear lines of communication with and responsibility to the organization's governance structures (such as the Board of Management) and be provided with a budget and approximate timeline for the completion of research. Membership, however, can be drawn from other local stakeholders, pro bono experts, colleagues from similar projects in other locations and so on. This group could be a significant resource subsequent to commissioning the research, offering guidance on methodology and dissemination and interpretation of findings, so it is worth giving the membership consideration. It is likely that the RFT will go through a number of drafts before being finalized, so allow time for this. It should, however, include the key elements presented in the following sections.

Background

Generally, the background will indicate who the commissioning agent is and the context for the research or evaluation. It might also indicate the experience of research in this community or organization to date and the implications of this.

Research focus

This section should outline exactly what is being evaluated, e.g. the specific programme of work or service being examined. It may outline what the commissioner wants to find out, including any specific questions to be answered.

Methodology

This section should present the expectations or preferences for research methods. If the methods to be used are open to negotiation, it is important to indicate this. If the organization is clear it is primarily interested in a particular type of evaluation, such as qualitative, narratives, etc., this should be specified. If the organization knows it is not interested in certain types of methodology, such as online surveys or case studies, state this also, with the rationale. Many researchers will see this clarity of expectation as a positive element of the invitation. This section will also indicate the tools or instruments to be used by the researchers. Standardized tools are those which are internationally accepted, tried and tested, and agreed as measuring what they set out to measure (Stewart, 1999). They can be expensive to use, as they often require a licence fee, and sometimes necessitate staff training. However, they enable data to be compared nationally and internationally, which can be extremely helpful, as well as having inherent credibility. Not all evaluations use standardized tools, but rather incorporate methods developed especially for the piece of work at hand (Stewart, 1999). This may save time and money, and could even feel like a more tailored approach, but it does bring limitations, particularly in relation to making valid comparisons with other studies, so it needs careful consideration.

Timelines

The proposed start dates, the suggested timelines for data collection, analysis, provision of interim and final reports and the completion of the work should be outlined. Space for receiving draft reports, providing feedback and receiving amended versions should be included.

Monitoring and accountability

The RFT should outline the mechanisms through which the researcher will be required to report on progress, issues arising, expenditure and so on. Suggested report headings are noted in Table 3.4 below, but there should also be an openness to creativity in how these reports are provided, especially if it is intended that they will be shared with non-traditional audiences. The RFT may suggest or welcome creative media such as blogs, social media, podcasts and so on. The monitoring and accountability processes should be based on effective communication between the researcher and commissioner. The frequency of anticipated meetings or informal engagement should be specified, as well a requirement for one named liaison person, as this can significantly help effective communication.

Minimum standards

There are some fundamental requirements worth stating in the RFT and again in the subsequent contract, for the avoidance of confusion. All documents should be spellchecked and proofread before submission to the commissioner. Minimum and maximum word counts should be specified and at least adhered to approximately. Full references must be included in a consistent

Table 3.4 Reporting templates

Progress Report Template	*Final Report Template*
• State of play • Practical difficulties/challenges and solutions • Methodology issues • Process evaluation • Current or future concerns • Important dates/timelines • Working arrangements • Finance report	• Executive summary • Introduction and Context • Methodology • Findings/Results • Discussion • Recommendations • Finance Report • Conclusion

manner. Some organizations will have specific requirements regarding writing style, e.g. font size, spacing, UK vs. US spellings, etc. These should be clearly stated from the outset.

Assessment and scoring process

It is important to consider and indicate how the submissions will be scored and what the process for shortlisting applicants is. The RFT should indicate any intention to interview and the timing and expected content of interviews. Key areas for assessment and scoring can include the team's qualifications, their experience of working in a similar community/with a similar target group, the expected costs and the team's ability to meet timelines. Also important to assess is the proposed methodology and fit with the organizational culture and any evidence of innovation, creative methods and tailored approaches. It is also important to assess the overall quality of the proposal. Whatever areas score submissions are to be made on, it will be necessary to ensure that the RFT document requests that applicants provide the relevant information, so these need to be cross-checked to ensure consistency before finalizing.

If the process will include conducting interviews with potential candidates, this will require an additional score sheet, on which the ultimate decision will be based. This may include assessments of the communication skills evidenced in the interview, assessments of flexibility, openness to collaboration, joint problem solving and understanding of the local context.

Having agreed the RFT and received approval from the appropriate governance structure, the working group will then need to circulate it according to the procurement thresholds outlined earlier. Utilizing existing networks is often the central mechanism for circulating the RFT and some relevant websites used by researchers were presented earlier in Table 3.1.

Understanding an RFT and making a submission

Before setting about fully understanding an RFT, the researcher makes a very rapid and crucial decision. The content is considered as relevant to the researcher or not, a check is made to see if information on the budget is available and, based on the costs and the area of expertise, a decision is made as to whether or not to pursue the request. Once the researcher has decided to proceed with a submission, the next task is to fully understand and interpret the RFT. One of the key components of a successful tender bid is the ability to understand and interpret not only what the commissioner requires but also what is needed in order for the finished project to be successful and to meet the client's needs. While some commissioners may know exactly what they want, not all will, and those who do know are often open to suggestions for improvement.

The first and foremost priority for a successful tender bid is to identify, clarify and confirm the key or overarching aim of the RFT. This may not always be straightforward, as commissioners may consist of organizations or committees with competing or conflicting priorities, needs and demands for budgets. Prior to the writing of the tender bid or indeed the identification of the key aim, it is important for the researcher to investigate and understand the structure and members of the commissioning body. One might ask what the commissioner's philosophy or management style is. Is the commissioner an individual or a committee from within an organization or a committee with members from different organizations with competing priorities but a common goal? Questions about who exactly the members of the commissioning body are and what their background is also need to be asked in order to understand the RFT. Once these questions have been answered, the researcher is then ready to try to understand and interpret the key aim of the RFT.

Knowing who the commissioner is helps the researcher to decide what exactly they want. RFTs may be as short as a single paragraph or may be a very comprehensive and detailed document. While it may seem obvious, it is necessary to read the RFT and continue to read and reread it throughout the writing process to ensure the response stays on track. The first reading should be a quick one to get an overall sense of the commissioners' requirements; this is followed by a more detailed reading with the reader highlighting what they believe to be the key points within the document. It is a good idea to have a second team member do the same independently of the first reader.

Once the key aim of the tender is decided upon, the researcher then sets about writing a submission. The commissioner may specify precisely the information required in an RFT response, and the researcher needs to know and be cognizant of the award criteria throughout the submission phase. This may include some or all of the following sections.

Introduction and background

The researcher needs to demonstrate that they are familiar with relevant policy documents, strategies and research already published in the area of study and should also know about any unpublished reports or previous studies that the commissioner may have undertaken.

Statement of the key aim and objectives

The researcher needs to state their understanding of the key aim or requirement of the RFT. The objectives should then be stated and these need to be specific, measurable, achievable, realistic and timely (Doran, 1981; Yemm, 2013).

Study design and methodology

The design of the study should be appropriate and match the objectives. The commissioner may have specified the design required within the RFT but the researcher can suggest an alternative if they believe it meets the requirements of the key aim more effectively. Including a rationale for the proposed change is important.

Data analysis and results

A data management and analysis plan needs to be proposed within the tender submission. This should be appropriate for the study design and methodology. The manner in which results will be reported should also be explored and this should be reflected in the outputs and deliverables. Tenderers can draw upon the excellent checklists available online and developed by a team of international experts for the analysis and reporting of varying study designs (e.g. http://strobe-statement.org/index.php?id=available-checklists).

Timeline of outputs and deliverables

A timeline of outputs and deliverables which reflect the design and the objectives should be provided. The researcher needs to commit to delivering specific targets to the commissioner throughout the study process. These may include: a detailed study protocol; ethical approval; agreement for access to services, industries or clients; progress reports; development and validation of a product, etc.

Project management and expertise

Clear details on the lines of accountability and reporting are required. Who within the research team will assume overall responsibility for the successful delivery of the tender? This is particularly important in joint and collaborative bids. The relevant expertise of the team members needs to be stated and this again should reflect the key aim, the objectives and the methodology chosen.

Ethics and good research practice

Ethical considerations need to be discussed and the implications ethical issues may have in terms of time and costs need to be stated.

Costing

If it is possible, the researcher should gain clarity on the budget in advance of making a submission. If this is not possible, the researcher must cost the work on the usual basis. However, it may be possible to provide the commissioner with a number of financial options.

Added value

Although it is not often explicitly asked, the researcher should consider what added value they can bring to the task. This is an opportunity for the researcher to highlight what they and their team can contribute over and above their competitors.

Throughout the writing of the submission, the researcher should be reflecting on the RFT, continuing to research the background of the commissioning agent and ensuring that their submission is easy to read, provides sufficient information on each of the awarding criteria and clearly meets the needs of the commissioner and not the researcher.

Communication and dissemination

As noted above, it is good practice to establish monitoring and oversight mechanisms from the outset of a tender process. Regular communication – both written and verbal – between the parties will be central to identifying difficulties early on, agreeing appropriate solutions and ensuring a common understanding of the task. Putting in place both formal and informal communication systems from the outset would prove helpful. Agreement regarding a hierarchy of documents, whereby agreed revisions to minutes, contracts, etc. replace older versions, will enable this principle to be effected in practice.

For the purposes of review, it is often helpful to separate out operational issues from strategic ones, although this will be impacted by the size of the budget, extent of the evaluation, time frame for completion and so on. If it is sensible to combine the structures to consider these elements, then they should at least be defined in terms of the meeting agenda. Operational issues that may require consideration include ensuring appropriate consent has been secured and, if not, how to encourage this, or how information is provided effectively to address any concerns. Participation by the target group may need to be monitored to ensure that the evaluation has an appropriate sample and if there are what can be done do to improve this. The researchers may need to consider whether there are other events in the community which should inform the data collection process.

The commissioning organization will need to think about appropriate methods and structures for monitoring progress and maintaining an overview of the work, and there are a number of options that can be considered. Monthly review meetings can allow the partners to consider progress and any operational issues, etc. This offers an opportunity for those directly engaged in fieldwork to get to know the commissioning organization and seek help and clarification if needed, and for the commissioner to help shape activities without influencing outcomes. Quarterly review meetings with the senior researchers and managers allow for the consideration of the overall focus of the work, issues arising, learning to date, possibilities for feedback loops, etc. These would generally be high level, strategic meetings. It can be effective to use standard reporting templates to indicate required information and reporting schedules. It is recommended that the commissioner provide a draft template for this, and agree its content prior to contractual sign off (see Table 3.4 for examples). Financial reports are central to effective monitoring of the progress. Again, it is important to specify what information is needed, how often and in what format. It should be borne in mind that research and academic institutions will have their own well-established financial reporting systems, and it may be easier to accept reports in the existing framework, whereas smaller organizations or independent consultants are more likely to be able to complete a template the commissioner provides them with. Either way, it is important to be clear about how expenditure should be broken down, e.g. salaries, travel and subsistence, licensing of standard tools, etc.

The negotiation process leading up to the finalization of a contract should include discussion about how emerging issues will be managed. As noted above, the importance of flexibility and being responsive to the community is vital, whilst also holding the integrity of the research process. In terms of reporting, this may take several forms, from detailed written reports to outline findings, verbal reports and audio visual reports. The reporting format will depend on the target audience and researchers may need to accommodate various needs within the commissioning organization.

Strategic issues which should be considered as the work progresses include identifying the emerging learning and considering who needs to be involved in interpreting this data. Communication should consider how to share lessons with the community and/or stakeholders, making this an explicit part of a dissemination plan. The issue of dissemination is considered in a number of later chapters in this text. Chapter 9 considers the sensitivities of sharing unexpected or potentially negative findings, and the implications for the researchers, while Chapter 10 explores the challenges of wider dissemination, including the impact of research on practice and policy.

Principles of ownership, intellectual property and data protection

Related to both the overall tendering, evaluation and reporting process is the issue of ownership of the work and intellectual property. These can be difficult to address retrospectively and should be considered in developing the RFT and finalizing the contract.

Ireland's Copyright and Related Rights Act (2000) has brought Irish law into conformity with all obligations incurred under international law on copyright and related rights. However, intellectual property rights (IPR) can differ from country to country, so on specific issues it is best to clarify with local legal advisors. IPR cover many different areas including patents, trademarks and copyrights. Research and evaluation data will fall under the field of copyright. An important point to clarify is that facts and ideas cannot be copyrighted. Only the form of expression in which facts and ideas are used can be protected. However, a compilation of facts which involves some creative input can generally be copyrighted.

The general rule in Ireland and elsewhere is that the person who creates/writes something owns it and has the right to exploit it (e.g. reproduce, sell, license, perform) and to prevent others from using it without consent. The creator also has the ability to transfer these rights to another. Simply paying someone to create something does not usually give the commissioner the right to exploit the creation; the creator must specifically assign those rights to the commissioner (European Commission, 2003).

Where an employee in the course of their contractual employment creates a work, the employer is the owner of the copyright of the work, unless an agreement to the contrary exists. However, this principle does not apply to an independent contractor or, generally, in the academic environment, unless agreed in advance. In the case of work specially ordered or commissioned, both parties must agree in writing that ownership lies with the commissioning entity or the assigned grantee. Joint ownership can also be agreed, and free use of the findings, report or other products is also possible, irrespective of who holds the copyright. The extent to which open access to and sharing of the findings will be encouraged is a very important but ultimately subjective decision.

There are a number of different mechanisms to protect intellectual property, depending on the product. These include patents, design registration, trademarks and copyright. For written work, including academic research, copyright is the appropriate way to protect intellectual property (see www.gov.uk/government/organisations/intellectual-property-office).

Drafting and implementing a copyright ownership and IPR policy is an important step in clarifying the relationship between commissioners of research and evaluation and those commissioned to undertake the work. IPR discussions can be a useful starting point in setting out the collaborative framework of the evaluation process between commissioners and evaluators and in managing data management issues generally. Indeed, the value of a professional approach to IPR, feeding into communication planning and to reporting, monitoring and accountability in general, is difficult to overstate.

Clarity at the beginning will help ensure the evaluation is initiated smoothly and minimize the possibilities of misunderstandings or disputes arising over the use and ownership of data. Key values that may be brought forward in mapping an IPR relationship include flexibility, centrality of relationships, negotiation, trust and clarity of expectations. There are various options available in negotiating IPR. These include one or other party having full and exclusive ownership. In general, this is not helpful, as it may not engender positive relationships and trust. Another possibility is that the commissioner owns all data and rights, whilst a license, subject to the necessary data protections (as discussed below), is provided to the evaluator to allow the data to be used for their own academic research, publication and/or other related educational purposes. However, as projects have evolved, further questions of ownership and rights may need to be clarified. For example, if the evaluator has the right to use the data, do they also have permission to manipulate it and use it in derivative works and for commercial purposes? Can they license others to use the data? If the information is made available in the public domain, can third parties freely use it for commercial purposes? The following are some key issues to be considered as part of an IPR review.

Awareness and sensitivity to IPR could be used in the scoring of submissions and further addressed at the interview stage. In the awarding and developing of the final contract, any particular concerns raised could be specifically addressed, following input and discussion with both parties and legal advice if necessary.

Clarity of ownership and use

The Irish Patents Office's *Good Practice Guide* recommends that "Contracts with employees or external consultants should have clear provisions on IPR ownership. Research institutions, for example, should have clear policies and agreements in place regarding researchers as well as students on ownership of IP [intellectual property] generated during their course of study, research and training" (European Commission, 2013). As noted above, the IPR policy should be stated at the Request for Tender stage. Some tender documents simply assert that "[Funding body] will retain all the intellectual property rights".

More sophisticated versions can assert arrangements along the following lines: "Copyright in all intellectual property developed under the contract will vest with [commissioner]. Licensing arrangements will be established to ensure that all materials and intellectual property are available to evaluators for academic and educational purposes. The evaluator agrees not to make commercial use of evaluation data without the permission of [commissioner]".

In developing the ownership model, it is important to clarify what parts of an evaluation a commissioner owns and does not own. For example, the researcher may own the report and the aggregate data but not the survey methodology or the questions used in the survey (even if developed as part of the evaluation project). In addition to making their own statement, the commissioners could request an IPR statement from potential researchers on their own IP policies, as well as highlighting previous experience in managing IP and data issues and identifying any particular IPR issues that might arise in the project tendered for and assessing how these would be managed.

One issue to be considered is whether the data will be a source of revenue. If so, scenarios in which researchers, commissioners and third parties benefit commercially from the research need to be clarified. It is conceivable that a funded project might be the springboard for a commercial project in the future and that a commissioner/researcher might want to maintain control over evaluation data for commercial purposes. An IPR policy should protect knowledge dissemination.

In considering dissemination, the parties should consider situations where the commissioner can control or prevent the distribution of data and/or an evaluation report. It is important to discuss expectations regarding an absolute right to publish and whether a licence would permit educational and government agencies to use the report free of charge. Similarly, it is important to consider permissions to use the report for non-commercial purposes. If the report has commercial value, it is important to consider a ratio of remuneration for the commissioner and the researcher.

As part of this process, it is important to explore whether third parties would be free to use the work for their own purposes or if it is better to approve each particular proposal as it arises. It is conceivable that a third party may use reports as the basis for commercial projects. In this situation, it is important to consider what limits, controls or licensing arrangements can be put in place to manage this. Finally, requirements regarding the citation of the parties must be considered, including whether there are circumstances in which credit will not be acknowledged (e.g. an author will generally be named when a publication is cited, but the organization that paid for a study might not). It might be possible or desirable to agree on how the credit is given, so as to increase the chance that all involved parties will be credited.

Data protection policy

Commissioners and researchers engaging directly with members of the public may require a data protection policy. Researchers who may be unfamiliar with the concept will benefit from clarification of their obligations in database management, and this should be an item for discussion at planning meetings. All participants must be clear about protecting data that could identify participants.

There are three main responsibilities in terms of obtaining data that both parties need to be aware of. Fair obtaining relates to making people aware of the uses of information gathered for the research or evaluation, for example, specifying whether consent has been obtained for any secondary uses of participants' data. Purpose specification requires that people are clear about the purpose (or purposes) for which personal information is kept. Parties to the process will need to assign responsibility for maintaining data sets. Finally, use and disclosure of information requires that there are defined rules about the use and disclosure of information and that individuals are aware of the uses and disclosures of their personal data. It is important to ensure that everyone understand the limitations in how individual data can be used.

Conclusion

This chapter aimed to provide guidance on the processes and procedures that can support and strengthen the relationships between those who commission research and evaluation and those who undertake it, with a specific focus on the early engagement and agreements reached between the parties. This is an area which is highly regulated and often shaped by legislation which aims to clarify issues of control and ownership, though it exists in a context which requires collaboration and responsiveness as highlighted in Chapter 2. The authors have set out processes that will hopefully enable the avoidance of legislative action and rather provide frameworks that enable key issues to be considered and agreed from the outset. This approach is underpinned by principles of transparency and respect rather than control and territorialism.

Inevitably, and as with all kinds of engagement, relationships between commissioners and grantees of research can be complex, and anticipating, minimizing and planning for conflict or, at the very least, differing priorities, can pay dividends as the work develops and issues emerge. Whilst there are regulations to inform procurement and contracting processes, best practice, common sense and good communication are likely to be key tools in establishing effective commissioning relationships.

Acknowledgements

The authors would like to thank the Department of Children and Youth Affairs in Ireland, and The Atlantic Philanthropies who supported much of the work referenced above.

References

Canavan, J., Coen, L., Ozan, J., & Curtin, C. (2014) *Leading community change: Delivering better outcomes in an Irish community. Childhood Development Initiative final process evaluation report*. Dublin: Childhood Development Initiative.

Comiskey, C.M. (2013) 'A three year national longitudinal study comparing drug treatment outcomes for opioid users with and without children in their custodial care and intake', *Journal of Substance Abuse Treatment*, 44, pp. 90–96.

Comiskey, C.M. & Snel, A. (2016) 'Using client's routine urinalysis records from multiple treatment systems to model five year opioid substitution treatment outcomes and improve the quality and usefulness of patient record management systems', *Substance Use and Misuse*, 51(12), pp. 1600–1609

Doran, G. (1981) 'There's a SMART way to write managements goals and objectives', *Management Review (AMA Forum)*, 70(11), pp. 35–36.

The European Commission (2003) *Intellectual property: Good practice guide* [Online]. Available from www.patentsoffice.ie/en/About-Us/IP-for-Business/Good-Practice-Guide.pdf (Accessed: 23 May 2017).

Government of Ireland (2000) *Copyright and related rights acts.* Available from www.irishstatutebook.ie/eli/2000/act/28/enacted/en/html

Irish Statute Book (2000) *Copyright and Related Rights Act* [Online]. Available from www.irishstatutebook.ie/eli/2000/act/28/enacted/en/pdf (Accessed: 23 May 2017).

McCawley, P.F. (2001) *The logic model for program planning and evaluation.* University of Idaho Extension. Available from www.uiles.uidaho.edu/extension/logicmodel.pdf (Accessed: 13 April 2011).

Meir, P.S., Donnell, M.C. & McElduff, P. (2004) 'Characteristics of drug users who do or do not have care of their children', *Addiction*, 99, pp. 955–961.

Murphy, T., MurphyA. and Smith, G., (2011) *Quality services, better outcomes.* Dublin: Childhood Development Initiative.

Office of the Revenue Commissioners (n.d.) *Research & development.* Available from www.revenue.ie/en/tax/ct/research-development.html (Accessed: 28 May 2017).

SoukeriahM., & Tannock, S., (2013). 'On the problem of over researched communities: The case of the Shatila Palestinian Refugee Camp in Lebanon', *Sociology*, 47(3), pp. 494–508.

Stewart, S. (1999). 'The use of standardised and non standardised assessments in a social services setting: Implications for practice', *British Journal of Occupational Therapy*, 62(9), pp. 417–423.

World Trade Organization (2014). *Government procurement agreement.* Signed in Israel: WTO.

Yemm, G. (2013) *Essential guide to leading your team: How to set goals, measure performance and reward talent.* Harlow: Pearson Education, pp. 37–39.

4 Governance and ethics in community-based research and evaluation

Sinéad McNally, Tara Murphy, Mark Morgan and Siobhán Keegan

Introduction

This chapter draws on current guidelines for the regulation of research practices to highlight governance and ethical implications for those commissioning and undertaking community-based research and evaluation. Increasingly, researchers are required by funders, research organizations and legislation to meet standards regarding research governance practices (Shaw et al., 2005; Banks et al., 2013). This shift towards external regulation of research is driven by a desire to ensure research integrity, whereby research is appropriate, transparent and effective, and has led to the development of research guidelines in most developed countries. Historically, research practices have been most strictly regulated in health research (e.g. clinical trials). However, research integrity is also of critical importance in research and evaluation of community-based programmes and interventions. As considered in detail in Chapter 2 of this text, community-based research and evaluation aims to respond to the needs of communities and lead to improved services and policies, and is driven by a respect for individuals in the community where community stakeholders are viewed as equal partners in the research process. Questionable research practice, or even research misconduct, in the form of insensitivity and/or incompetence on the part of the researcher may have unintended negative consequences for community stakeholders (Bamberger et al., 2012) and mechanisms for minimizing such practices must be considered early by those commissioning and conducting community-based research and evaluation.

To maintain research integrity, good research governance is essential. Research governance is "the system of administration and supervision through which research is managed, participants and staff are protected, and accountability is assured" (Shaw, Boynton & Greenhalgh, 2005, p. 497). As highlighted by Shaw et al., it is not conceived of as the responsibility of any single entity but rather as something that is relevant for everyone (Shaw et al., 2005). Good research governance will ensure that systems are in place so that research is (1) ethical, (2) well founded with a clear rationale, (3) disseminated openly and (4) managed responsibly in terms of data protection and financial management.

This chapter begins by considering expectations for research governance in an international context. The extent to which researchers are required to follow specific guidelines with regard to research governance varies internationally and across disciplines. For example, the UK government moved towards implementing a centralized system for research governance for health and social care research ahead of other countries such as Australia (National Health and Medical Research Council) and the United States of America (Code of Federal Regulations, Department of Health and Human Services). This centralized system is referred to as the Research Governance Framework (RGF) for health and social care research and will be discussed further in relation to international standards for research governance and ethics. Although the RGF is of direct relevance for health and social care, it offers general principles of good practice and is intended to be relevant for any research where "poor practice could have a direct impact on the health or wellbeing of the public" (Department of Health, 2005).

Variability in governance and regulation in different settings and jurisdictions can create challenges for research and evaluation conducted in a community setting. However, all researchers are bound by professional codes of practice such as the Declaration of Helsinki (Shaw et al., 2005) to conduct research in an ethical and responsible manner. This chapter will therefore also consider the work of research ethics committees (RECs), also known as institutional review boards (IRBs), and their basic remit as part of good research governance. The process for evaluating proposals for ethics approval is outlined, including a set of questions that are useful for the researcher in guiding the development of a detailed and well-thought-out proposal for community-based research and evaluation. The chapter concludes with a special focus on obtaining informed consent and considers the ethical challenges facing commissioners and researchers with regard to this key ethical issue.

Research governance: International context

Research regulation and governance guidelines vary internationally. In the UK, the Research Governance Framework (RGF) for healthcare research sets out five key standards and responsibilities for good research practice: (1) ethics – with respect to participant rights, dignity, respect and due diligence; (2) science – providing a clear rationale for the research and chosen methodology; (3) information – making dissemination of research findings open and transparent; (4) health, safety and employment – following NHS guidelines; and (5) finance and intellectual property – appropriate management of budgets and data (Howarth & Kneafsey, 2005). As a result, those intending to undertake research (including clinicians) are required to seek both ethical and research governance approval prior to commencing their research (Fontenla & Rycroft-Malone, 2006; Howarth, Kneafsey, & Haigh, 2008). In effect, the RGF aims to ensure that all health and social care research is aligned to best research practice in terms of ethics, robustness, quality and cost effectiveness. For research that falls outside the remit of the RGF, researchers must look to other regulatory bodies. Non-clinical research conducted in a community setting must meet research standards as set out by the organization to which the researcher belongs. UK universities have signed the Concordat to Support Research Integrity which was developed by Universities UK (UUK) in collaboration with the Higher Education Funding Council for England (HEFCE), Research Councils UK (RCUK) and the Wellcome Trust. It identifies five principles by which universities are expected to engage in research: (1) with rigour and integrity; (2) with appropriate ethical, legal and professional obligations and standards; (3) with good governance and a culture of integrity; (4) with transparency and fairness regarding allegations of research misconduct; and (5) an open and regular review of progress made (Universities UK, 2012).

Centralization of review systems appears to occur in smaller countries (e.g. the UK, Denmark and New Zealand) or is often only for one sector (e.g. health) or type of research (e.g. clinical trials). In both the US and Canada, clinical research is regulated by nationally coordinated ethics committees (Shaw et al., 2005). Canada's Research Ethics Boards review and approve research protocols, and the Canadian Institutes for Research regulate research conduct. Canadian policy states that all disciplines should share certain ethical standards and principles when conducting research with human participants, and these principles are articulated in the Tri-Council Policy Statement (Canadian Institutes, 2014). In the US, research with any human participants must be reviewed by IRBs, and research conduct is regulated by the US Office for Human Research Protections.

In keeping with other countries, review systems for health and clinical trial research in Ireland have greater visibility than review systems for other types of research. The Clinical Trials Committee regulates clinical RECs, but there is no centralized overview or regulation of other types of REC. In general, RECs are less prominent in Ireland than in other English-speaking countries (Felzmann, Sixsmith, O'Higgins, Ni Chonnachtaigh, & Nic Gabhainn, 2010). However, there have been significant developments with regard to regulating research governance and ethics in the academic sector, and the following section considers the implications of such developments for community-based research and evaluation.

Research governance in a community setting

In requiring researchers to be accountable for the way in which their research is conducted, appropriate governance systems will ensure that research is transparent and based on best available knowledge and that funding is managed responsibly (i.e. that it is relevant and has usable outputs). However, implementing required standards of research governance can be quite challenging when conducting community-based research and evaluation (Banks et al., 2013). At times, seemingly unnecessary or overly demanding requirements may hinder rather than help the research process, and may place time and financial burdens on the researcher, especially if they have not encountered such systems previously. In addition to potential time and cost burdens, researchers and commissioners of research may stop looking at important ethical issues that are unique to researching in a community context because they are overly focused on fulfilling requirements as set out by the Research Ethics Committee (REC), for example. It is important that the researcher and those commissioning research, including the community with whom the programmes are being developed and delivered, are engaged in the ethics and governance process so that all parties are not relying on the ethics committee to identify potential ethical challenges. This is especially so in community-based research where there may also be

> Specific issues relating to the ethics of partnership working, collaboration, blurring of boundaries between researchers and researched, community rights, community conflict and democratic participation.
>
> (Banks et al., 2013, p. 263, when discussing ethical issues unique to community-based participatory research)

In an evaluation of the Research Governance Framework (RGF) across fourteen primary care organizations, Howarth et al. (2008) found that a significant proportion of researchers (n=36, 47%) experienced the research management procedures as being unhelpful, frustrating or obstructive. Researchers proposed several reasons for this, including the delay in seeking criminal background checks as well as the lengthy ethics application processes. Previous research by Leese et al. (2005) and later Gerrish & Guillaume (2006) highlighted a delay in conducting multi-site and cross-border studies which may require ethical approval from multiple ethics committees. Gerrish and Guillaume (2006) found that the time to gain ethical approval from the National Health Service (NHS) REC ranged from ten to thirty-eight weeks.

Thompson and France (2010) highlighted the ongoing challenges in undertaking clinical research under the auspices of the NHS. Though their experience of seeking ethical approval was generally positive, they were keen to emphasize the difficulty in overcoming the requirements for Research Management and Governance approval (or R&D approval as it is more commonly referred to) which can involve seeking approval from a large number of trusts and services (Thompson & France, 2010). In their study of the research governance process in which they sought trust management approval in England and Scotland, Thompson and France's (2010) timeline for recruitment and data collection had been delayed by four months, which required an extension of their study and additional funding and impacted on key deliverables. In this case, neither the funder nor the researcher had any managerial control in the research management and governance procedures of the various trusts or services (Thompson & France, 2010).

Research governance and ethical processes are implemented to protect the safety and wellbeing of participants as well as to promote transparency and accountability (Howarth et al., 2008). While necessary, the parameters arising from such processes may prove administratively burdensome for researchers undertaking community-based or real-world research. As is discussed extensively throughout this book, community-based research must account for and respond to the priorities and expectations of multiple stakeholders, historical and cultural factors, health and social care issues, local policies, relationships, champions and so on. Add to this the governance structure of the funder (potentially a management committee, scientific or expert advisory group or an implementation support group) and one begins to wonder, '*What's in it for the researcher?*' given that so much of this is out of their control and yet is likely to determine the success or failure of the research.

The desire to ensure research integrity and minimize social harm requires balancing safety measures and bureaucracy (Lunt & Fouché, 2010). Beyond governance guidelines and regulations, tension can arise in real world studies where there is a mismatch between the priorities and expectations of commissioners and researchers. For example, combined evaluation and implementation of a child or family intervention can cause tension for staff, who are concerned with the daily delivery of the intervention, and researchers, who are primarily concerned with measuring the efficacy and effectiveness of the intervention and ultimately with producing knowledge that it publishable. It is therefore imperative that researchers and commissioners seek early clarification regarding the roles, responsibilities and expectations of both parties. In other words, making the implicit 'explicit' is important in order to safeguard the smooth undertaking of the research study. An adequate research governance framework has the potential to promote and enhance the quality and integrity of the research. Good governance and ethics processes can maximize resources, avoid duplication, minimize research fatigue and ultimately lead to a culture of scientifically rigorous and user-focused research.

Research ethics applications take time and the frequency with which committees meet will vary across organizations. Additional time should be allocated to preparing a submission, waiting for approval, revising an ethics application based on feedback and repeating the process. Unless time has been factored in for the ethical review process, delay in getting approval could prove costly in terms of additional salary and materials requirements. Costs may be especially high for research conducted across several sites and jurisdictions if governance structures are not identified at the planning stage and adequate preparations are not made for ethical submissions (Larson, Bratts, Zwanziger & Stone, 2004). The unpredictability of the ethics review process can also pose problems (Edwards, Stone & Swift, 2007). Often researchers and reviewers have different expectations of the design and methodology of the research project. This may be particularly so with regard to the use of qualitative research designs which may be developed with a significantly different view of the nature of research (Tilley, Powick-Kumar & Ratkovic, 2009; Lincoln & Tierney, 2004). However, there have been considerable developments with regard to understanding and examining ethical issues in qualitative research, e.g. the most recent editions of the *Canadian Tri-Council Policy Statement: Ethical Conduct for Research Involving Humans* (2010; 2014) include a chapter dedicated to ethical considerations for qualitative research (Canadian Institutes, 2014, Chapter 10).

Where differences of opinion arise, debate can be an important part of research and is an inherent part of ethical review, reflecting real engagement with the purpose and design of research and the benefits and risks for the participants (Autti-Rämö & Mäkelä, 2007; Felzmann et al., 2010). Nonetheless, division or conflict may be the natural outcome of stretching medical ethical review processes to fit social science research in a community setting (Pritchard, 2002; van den Hoonaard, 2002; Tilley et al., 2009). Social science research is likely to use different methodological approaches and conceptual frameworks (e.g. participatory research), and greater communication and training for those reviewing these research proposals is likely to be necessary to explore the particular challenges this type of research faces (Connolly & Reid, 2007). Ethical review will also depend on the research population (for example, see Felzmann et al. (2010) for a detailed consideration of the ethical review process for research involving children in Ireland). The following section considers in detail the role of the REC (or institutional review board (IRB)) in research governance and important considerations for those commissioning and conducting research in community settings.

Key ethics considerations in community-based research and evaluation

In Ireland and the United Kingdom, RECs are typically responsible for ethical review for social science research and evaluation. They are found in different settings, including the voluntary or community sector. In 2010 there were twenty-seven academic RECs on record in Ireland, the majority of which were central committees (Felzmann et al., 2010). Government or other funding bodies may focus on reviewing specially commissioned research with vulnerable populations in their care or recipients of their services, and may therefore have a specially commissioned REC. Operational guidelines for RECs, developed by the World Health Organization (WHO, 2000), specify that REC members must have relevant expertise and diversity, and that community membership is important. However, community membership is often limited in Ireland, which may negatively impact on community ownership and buy-in for research (Felzmann et al., 2010).

To submit a proposal to the REC, applicants typically complete an application form, providing any requested supporting documentation such as a detailed project description, information sheets and consent forms for participants. Submissions may: (1) be approved outright; (2) receive provisional approval pending minor amendments (the most frequent outcome); (3) be recommended for resubmission pending major revisions; or rejected outright (the rarest outcome) (ICB, 2004; NRES, 2007 in Felzmann et al., 2010). In all cases, researchers need to submit a detailed research proposal which includes the central research question, details and justification of the research methodology, plans for disseminating research findings, the target audience for the research, any potential conflicts of interest for the researcher and commissioner of the research and potential risks to the participants.

Key aspects of the application include details of sampling methods and how the researcher plans to inform participants about the nature of the research and the risks and benefits of that research, and to debrief them once the research is concluded. This information is an important part of the process of getting informed consent, as participants can only be considered to give informed consent once they have specific details about the research. In addition to the nature of the research and the potential risks that can be involved, participants need to know how long the research will take and plans for archiving or reusing the data, and they need to be informed that anonymity will be ensured, that participation is voluntary and that they can withdraw from the study at any time. In order to assess whether necessary measures are in place to facilitate participants' rights to anonymity and withdrawal from the study, researchers need to provide an information sheet and consent form. They also need to detail the practical steps they will take to ensure anonymization of the data, and how and for how long data will be stored and used.

Researchers' responsibilities for good ethical conduct

The researcher is responsible for the "protection of participants' rights, safety, and welfare, and for scientific integrity" (Merritt et al., 2010, p. 1). This has implications for the nature and quality of training delivered to fieldworkers so that they maintain good research practice. Fieldworkers are similarly responsible for undertaking fieldwork in an ethical manner that requires them to have a sufficient understanding of key ethical concepts such as 'informed consent', 'confidentiality', 'anonymity' and 'voluntary participation'.

There are no known standardized procedure(s) for educating or training fieldworkers to undertake research, particularly with vulnerable groups such as children, individuals with disabilities, elderly people and ethnic minorities. This is surprising given the level of responsibility assigned to fieldworkers in terms of engaging with participants and collecting data as well as the potential for challenges to occur in the real world. Researchers may be guided by certain research principles or a code of ethics as set out by their own academic institutions or professional bodies. These ethical codes may provide some assistance when addressing important ethical concepts with their fieldworkers.

For example, several internationally relevant codes of ethics have been developed in relation to conducting research with human participants. The British Psychological Society's (BPS) *Professional Code of Ethics* (2009) and the American Psychological Association's (APA) *Ethical Principles of Psychologists and Code of Ethics* (2010) aim to avoid or minimize any harm to participants (and equally to those gathering the data) arising from their participation in research. Both ethics codes address a range of key ethical issues, including informed consent, privacy and confidentiality, avoidance of harm, continuity of care and voluntary participation. The BPS sets out specific guidelines for research with children aged less than sixteen years, persons lacking capacity and individuals in a dependent or unequal relationship, and for dealing with sensitive topics such as participants' sexual behaviour, gender or experience of violence. The APA also provides guidelines for gaining informed consent for the recording of voices and images in research, the limits of confidentiality and the situation of multiple relations (e.g. where the researcher/psychologist may have a dual relationship with a participant). In addition, the *Australasian Code of Ethics for Direct Support Professionals* (Australasian Society for the Study of Intellectual Disability & McVilly, 2007) highlights the importance of performing your role within the limits of your capacity or expertise.

Similarly, the Irish Council for Bioethics (ICB) developed a set of recommendations for promoting research integrity (2010) which includes providing education and training to researchers in good research practice through the delivery of didactic teaching modules and mentoring by more senior researchers. Included in this definition of research misconduct is the fabrication, falsification and plagiarizing of results and ideas (ICB, 2010). *The Ethical Guidelines for Research with People with Disabilities* (National Disability Authority, 2009) (NDA) highlights the need to develop research processes that engage individuals with disabilities in an inclusive and meaningful way. The NDA (2009) suggests some practical things researchers can do in order to promote inclusivity of research participants including (p. 30):

- preparing large-print materials for participants with visual impairments;
- providing material in easy-to-read format for participants with intellectual disabilities;
- conducting interviews in venues that are accessible and safe;
- choosing a location for interviews to ensure not only accessibility and safety but also confidentiality;
- accommodating participants' physical needs, including access to the venue, comfort, care or refreshment breaks during the interviews/assessment period;
- providing appropriate disability awareness training for interviewers;
- accommodating any specific information and communication needs related to disability, including those related to speech, hearing, sight or cognitive impairment.

While these guidelines have been developed specifically for conducting research with people with disabilities, they are also applicable to undertaking research with other groups. In Ireland, all adults have a duty of care to children (and other vulnerable groups) as set out by the national guidelines for the protection and welfare of children (Department of Children and Youth

Affairs, 2011). For example, researchers who may witness a harmful act involving a child or young person have a duty of care to report the incident or observation to a higher authority, who should follow their organization's child protection policy. Fieldworkers for example should first report to the lead researcher who should then follow their ethical or child protection procedures. Obtaining written consent from parents or guardians is a legal requirement in countries such as Australia and Iceland (Dockett & Perry, 2007). Furthermore, consent should also be sought for using photos or videos in publications, contacting participants at a later stage as part of a longitudinal study and archiving data for future use by other bona fide researchers.

Obtaining informed consent

Perhaps the ethical issue that attracts the greatest attention when preparing a research proposal for ethics review is the process of gaining informed consent for research (Felzmann et al., 2010). To achieve informed consent, participants must receive adequate information on the intended research or evaluation project. In particular, participants must be informed that participation is voluntary, and they must be told about the proposed length of time involved, any potential risks of participating in the research, how data will be used and whether or not incentives are given for participation. Participants must also be informed about how the researcher and those commissioning research intend to store the data and whether it will be used again at a later date and/or shared with other researchers. Ensuring informed consent and anonymity for participants may be particularly challenging with unique participant groups such as children and young adults.

However, while gaining informed consent from children may be challenging, it is also important to recognize that in accordance with the UN Convention on the Rights of the Child, children have rights and responsibilities appropriate to their age, stage of development and culture. In line with this perspective, the *National Children's Strategy* (Department of Health and Children, 2000) proposes the need for children to be facilitated in participating in research in a way that is meaningful to them. One approach that has been developed to facilitate this process is the Mosaic approach, which has been developed with three- to four-year-old children in mind (Clarke & Moss, 2011). This approach is a way of involving children that acknowledges them as integrating their perspective with that of adults: it combines a verbal and visual approach and may involve drawings and photographs as well as observations, maps and interviews to access children's perspectives, awareness and understanding of the topic being investigated.

As noted above, the decisions made by RECs are intended to protect the wellbeing of participants, especially when sensitive issues are being considered or when the target population is considered vulnerable. A related debate centres on the question as to whether consent should be actively or passively sought (Range, Embry & McLeod, 2001). There is considerable variation in the type of personal or parental consent required in studies using participants considered to be particularly vulnerable. Even in countries with well-developed guidelines, there are differences depending on the sponsors of the research, with some requiring the parent or guardian of a minor to signify their permission in writing (i.e. active consent). In contrast, with passive consent a letter is sent to the parents of the participants explaining the nature of the study and giving the parent an opportunity to opt out of the study. However, a key feature of this procedure is that it is assumed that the young person will participate unless the parent takes action to withdraw from the study. While passive consent was traditionally the most common approach required by ethics committees, the experience of recent years suggests that some now require active consent (Higgerson et al., 2014). As will be evident from the research considered here, such a decision has important implications.

Significant challenges to the research project arise from using active consent procedures. The first is that the response rate is substantially lower than with passive consent procedures (Ellickson & Hawes, 1989). Sometimes the differences can be substantial; passive consent rates can be over 90 per cent, while active consent rates over 60 per cent are difficult to achieve. Furthermore, active parental consent can result in the underrepresentation of certain groups, including minorities, low achievers and young people who are at risk of engaging in problem behaviour (Ellickson & Hawes, 1989). This in turn limits the generalizability of the findings of the studies.

A study by Pokorny et al. (2001) examined the question of whether the response profiles obtained through active and passive consent are actually different with respect to substance use when that is the focus of the study. In their study in Chicago the passive consent procedure resulted in participation rates of 89 per cent, while the corresponding rate with active consent yielded a response rate of 55 per cent. Not only were there significant demographic differences between the two groups (particularly in terms of employment status), but they also differed with regard to substance use, particularly cigarette smoking. The authors concluded that the reliance on active consent procedures would therefore have led to an underestimation of the prevalence of smoking in this population. More recently, Courser et al. (2009) carried out an experimental study of forms of consent in fourteen Kentucky school districts. Half of the districts were randomly assigned to implement the survey of substance use with active consent procedures, while the other districts implemented the survey using passive consent procedures. In line with earlier work, they found substantial differences in participation rates, and in addition found that active consent procedures resulted in an overrepresentation of female students as well as older students. More importantly, the active consent group had lower rates of prevalence for most drugs as well as for most anti-social behaviours.

Not only are there differences between active and passive consent procedures, but the precise specifications of the procedure adopted can influence response rates. If parental consent is required, then the main options are by means of mail returns or through student-delivered forms. While RECs may opt for one of these on the basis of intuition or convenience, there is evidence that the approach taken makes a substantial difference. A study by McMorris et al. (2004) examined the returns (based on an active consent procedure) in a 'mail condition' whereby consent forms were returned by students to their classrooms, in a randomized control design in the Washington, DC, area. The results indicated a higher rate of return as well as agreement by parents to have their children in the study in the condition where students delivered the form to the classroom. While this study illustrates the possible impact of the details of the decision of an ethics committee, care should be taken in generalizing the particular results of that study to other cultural contexts. In conducting research with schools, one of the authors observed the significant administrative burdens which some schools experience. Research which places additional demands on schools may impact the likelihood of gaining the cooperation of schools, which is a critical matter in collecting data in school-going populations. Active procedures are likely to involve a school in more administration, especially if there is a requirement to collect the consent forms. In addition to carefully considering the way in which consent is achieved, researchers must also carefully consider the wording of research questions for younger participants, especially on sensitive questions, as this will impact the rate of response and quality of the data (Grube & Morgan, 1986). Overall, gaining informed consent highlights the need to consider not only the immediate research governance systems in the researcher's institution, but also the role of important stakeholders participating in or facilitating the research.

Obtaining meaningful assent

As previously discussed, most ethical guidelines require that adults provide written consent for their research participation or that parents provide written consent for their child's participation. However, in many cases there is no formally stated requirement for assent. Assent differs from consent and can be defined as affirmation to participate in research (Broome & Stieglitz, 1992). It also pre-supposes discussion of the research content, disclosure of any caveats and respect of the participants' rights and opinions. The fact that assent is often not required by law or explicitly required by ethics committees or research boards (Lindeke, Hauck & Tanner, 2000) means that it can sometimes be airbrushed out of the fieldwork process. The eliding of this seemingly obvious step may have the inevitable consequence that a lot of research happens without participants being fully informed about the research and their rights in relation to it.

The act of obtaining meaningful assent means that children and vulnerable adults possess a veto over their participation, regardless of whether a parent or guardian has consented to their participation (Broome & Stieglitz, 1992). Participant opinions and understanding of the research should be solicited to ensure that they attach accurate perceptions to the research content. Pedersen and Harbaugh (1995) reported that one of their child participants in a study of cardiac catheterization mistakenly thought that an overhead lamp was going to be used in the process. In the evaluation of an early childhood care and education programme, one of the authors of this chapter found that a five-year-old child became upset before a cognitive assessment took place in his primary school. He mistakenly thought that the researcher was going to administer an inoculation injection because the same room had been previously used for this purpose by a visiting doctor.

Danby and Farrell (2005) have commented that the notion of child assent is a relatively new one, which has meant that even if studies report that direct child assent was sought, readers have little knowledge of the process of engagement that leads up to assent being gained. In the case of older children (eight years and older) and adults, assent involves explaining the research, providing documentation, assuring confidentiality (with caveats if they exist), allowing time for discussion and asking if they are happy to take part, while also emphasizing that they have the right to stop or withdraw at any time. For younger children, it can be useful to ask the child's caregiver to list some information on the child's likes and interests before the research begins so that these topics can be used in initial conversations to engage with the child. Younger children are often likely to engage with and encode their world visually rather than verbally (Conrad, 1971; Hagen, Jongeward & Kail, 1975). It is also, therefore, best to 'show' a younger child or an adult with verbal comprehension difficulties what is in store rather than to tell them. Giving participants a chance to touch, handle and see the materials that will be used in the research is advisable before discussion about proceeding with the research.

The growing imperative to collect a representatively large sample of data quickly can mean that fieldworkers are often put in the position where, due to inadequate research funding or timelines, meaningful assent becomes an ideal world concept rather than an actuality. It is important for fieldworkers to resist the urge to collect data at any cost (Tinson, 2009). Funders and grant holders can help by designing and funding research that allows for the time to be taken to ensure that such assent is gained and to recruit alternative participants if it is not.

Conclusion

Good governance and a solid grasp of ethical considerations in real-world research and evaluation are critical to ensure usable and well-managed research that respects the rights and expectations of community participants and commissioners of research. While governance guidelines for clinical research are well developed and strictly implemented in most developed countries, governance requirements in the social sciences are more varied and often need to include different considerations regarding methodologies and conceptual approaches (e.g. qualitative methods and participatory research). Despite challenges involved in governance requirements for social science real-world research, ethical review is an integral part of research in this context, and all efforts should be made by the researcher and those commissioning research to implement transparent and effective research governance.

As ethical review in community-based research and evaluation often involves stretching medical ethical guidelines to new contexts, there is an ongoing need for debate and additional reflection in the ethical review process. This is especially so in community-based research and evaluation, where novel methodologies may be developed to more adequately research the experiences and needs of participants. The importance of debate in ethics is evident when debating the appropriateness of the types of, and ways in which, informed consent is obtained. Rather than shying away from debate on the appropriateness of particular methods and design, researchers and commissioners are encouraged to engage proactively with the ethical review process. In this way, new considerations may be discovered that would otherwise go unnoticed if trying to hurry through the ethical review process.

References

American Psychological Association (APA) (2010) *Ethical principles of psychologists and code of conduct*. Amended version of 2002*APA code of ethics.*

Australasian Society for the Study of Intellectual Disability & McVilly, K.R. (2007). *Australasian code of ethics for direct support professionals.* 1st edn. Rosanna, Vic.: Australasian Society for the Study of Intellectual Disability.

Autti-Rämö, I. & Mäkelä, M. (2007) 'Ethical evaluation in health technology assessment reports: An eclectic approach', *International Journal of Technology Assessment in Health Care*, 23(1), pp. 1–8. doi:10.1017/S0266462307051501

Bamberger, M., Rugh, J. & Mabry, L. (2012) *Real world evaluation: Working under budget, time, data, and political constraints.* 2nd edn. London: SAGE.

Banks, S., Armstrong, A., Carter, K., Graham, H., Hayward, P., Henry, A., Holland, T., Holmes, C., Lee, A., McNulty, A., Moore, N., Nayling, N., Stokoe, A. & Strachan, A. (2013) 'Everyday ethics in community-based participatory research', *Contemporary Social Science*, 8(3), pp. 263–277.

British Psychological Society (BPS) (2009) *Code of ethics and conduct: Guidance published by the Ethics Committee of the British Psychological Society.* Leicester: The British Psychological Society.

Broome, M.E. & Stieglitz, K.A. (1992) 'The consent process and children', *Research in Nursing & Health*, 15(2), pp. 147–152.

Canadian Institutes of Health Research, Natural Sciences and Engineering Research Council of Canada, Social Sciences and Humanities Research Council of Canada (2014) *Tri-council policy statement: Ethical conduct for research involving humans.* Ottawa, Canada.

Canadian Institutes of Health Research, Natural Sciences and Engineering Research Council of Canada, Social Sciences and Humanities Research Council of Canada (2010) *Tri-council policy statement: Ethical conduct for research involving humans.* Ottawa, Canada.

Clarke, A. & Moss, P. (2011) *Listening to children: The mosaic approach*. London: National Children's Bureau.

Connolly, K. & Reid, A. (2007) 'Ethics review for qualitative research: Adopting a values-based, facilitative approach', *Qualitative Inquiry*, 13(7), pp. 1031–1047.

Conrad, R. (1971) 'The chronology of the development of covert speech in children', *Developmental Psychology*, 5(3), p. 398.

Courser, M.W., Shamblen, S.R., Lavrakas, P.J., Collins, D. & Ditterline, P. (2009) 'The impact of active consent procedures on non-response and response error in youth survey data', *Evaluation Review*, 33, pp. 270–395.

Danby, S. & Farrell, A. (2005) 'Opening the research conversation', in Farrell, A. (ed) *Ethical research with children*. Milton Keynes: Open University Press, pp. 49–67.

Department of Children and Youth Affairs (2011) *Children first: National guidelines on the protection and welfare of children*. Dublin: Government Publications.

Department of Health and Children (Department of Children and Youth Affairs) (2000) *National children's strategy: Our children – their lives*. Dublin: The Stationery Office.

Department of Health (2001, 2005) *Research governance framework for health and social care*. London: Department of Health.

Dockett, S. & Perry, B. (2007) 'Trusting children's accounts in research', *Journal of Early Childhood Research*, 5(1), pp. 47–63.

Edwards, S., Stone, T. & Swift, T. (2007) 'Differences between research ethics committees', *International Journal of Technology Assessment in Health Care*, 23(1), pp. 17–23.

Ellickson, P.L. & Hawes, J.A. (1989) 'An assessment of active versus passive methods for obtaining parental consent', *Evaluation Review*, 13, pp. 45–55.

Felzmann, H., Sixsmith, J., O'Higgins, S., Ni Chonnachtaigh, S. & Nic Gabhainn, S. (2010) *Ethical review and children's research in Ireland*. Dublin: Office of the Minister for Children and Youth Affairs.

Fontenla, M. & Rycroft-Malone, J. (2006) 'Research governance and ethics: A resource for novice researchers', *Nursing Standard*, 20(23), pp. 41–46.

Gerrish, K. & Guillaume, L. (2006) 'Whither survey research: the challenges of undertaking postal surveys within the UK research governance framework', *Journal of Nursing Research*, 11, pp. 485–497.

Grube, J.W. & Morgan, M. (1986) *Smoking, drinking and other drug use among Dublin post-primary school pupils*. Dublin: Economic and Social Research Institute (General Publications).

Hagen, J.W., Jongeward, R.H. & Kail, R.V. (1975) 'Cognitive perspectives on the development of memory', *Advances in Child Development and Behavior*, 10, pp. 57–101.

Higgerson, R., Olsho, L., Christie, L.M., Rehder, K., Doksum, T., Gedeit, R., Giuliano, J.S., Brennan, B., Wendlandt, R. & Randolph, A.G. (2014) 'Variability in IRBs regarding parental acceptance of passive consent', *Pediatrics*, 134(2), pp. e496–e503.

Howarth, M.L. & Kneafsey, R. (2005) 'The impact of research governance in healthcare and higher education organizations', *Journal of Advanced Nursing*, 49, 675–683.

Howarth, M.L., Kneafsey, R. & Haigh, C. (2008) 'Centralization and research governance: does it work?' *Journal of Advanced Nursing*, 61(4), pp. 363–372.

Irish Council for Bioethics (ICB) (2010) *Recommendations for promoting research integrity*. Dublin: Irish Council for Bioethics.

Irish Council for Bioethics (ICB) (2004) *Operational procedures for research ethics committees: Guidance 2004*. Dublin: Irish Council for Bioethics.

Larson, E., Bratts, T., Zwanziger, J., & Stone, P. (2004) 'A survey of IRB process in 68 U.S. hospitals', *Journal of Nursing Scholarship*, 36, pp. 260–264.

Leese, G., Storey, C., Ford, J. & Cheater F. (2005) 'Researchers' responses to research management and governance for primary care research in England: Persistent and escalating problems over time', *Journal of Health Organisation & Management*, 19(6), pp. 494–503.

Lincoln, Y.S. & Tierney, W.G. (2004) 'Qualitative research and institutional review boards', *Qualitative Inquiry*, 10, pp. 219–234.

Lindeke, L.L., Hauck, M.R. & Tanner, M. (2000) 'Practical issues in obtaining child assent for research', *Journal of Pediatric Nursing*, 15(2), pp. 99–104.

Lunt, N. & Fouché (2010) 'Practitioner research, ethics and research governance', *Ethics and Social Welfare*, 4(3), pp. 219–235.

McMorris, B.J., Clements, J., Evans-Whipp, T., Gangnes, D., Bond, L. & Toumbourou, J.W. (2004) 'A comparison of methods to obtain active parental consent for an international survey', *Evaluation Review*, 28, pp. 64–83.

Merritt, M.W., Labrique, A.B., Katz, J., Rashid, M., West, K.P. Jr. & Pettit, J. (2010) 'A field training guide for human subjects research ethics', *PLoS Medicine*, 7(10), p. e1000349.

National Disability Authority (NDA) (2009) *Ethical guidance for research with people with disabilities.* Dublin: National Disability Authority.

National Research Ethics Service (2007) *Standard operating procedures for research ethics committees in the United Kingdom.* Version 3.4. London: National Research Ethics Service.

Pederson, C. & Harbaugh, B.L. (1995) 'Children's and adolescents' experiences while undergoing cardiac catheterization', *Maternal-child Nursing Journal*, 23, pp. 15–25.

Pokorny, S.B., Jason, L.A., Schoeny, M.E., Townsend, S.M. & Curie, C.J. (2001) 'Do participation rates changes when active consent procedures replace passive consent', *Evaluation Review*, 25, pp. 567–580.

Pritchard, I.A. (2002) 'Travelers and trolls: Practitioner research and institutional review boards', *Educational Researcher*, 31(3), pp. 3–13.

Range, L., Embry, T. & MacLeod, T. (2001) 'Active and passive consent: a comparison of actual research with children', *Ethical Human Sciences and Services*, 3(1), pp. 23–31.

Shaw, S., Boynton, P.M. & Greenhalgh, T. (2005) 'Research governance: where did it come from? What does it mean?', *Journal of the Royal Society of Medicine*, 98(11), pp. 496–502.

Shaw, S., Macfarlane, F., Carter, Y.H. & Letley, L. (2005) 'Developing primary care research teams: a qualitative interview study in UK general practice', *Australian Journal of Primary Health*, 11, pp. 24–31.

Thompson, A.G.H. & France, E.F. (2010) 'One stop or full stop? The continuing challenges for researchers despite the new streamlined NHS research governance process', *BMC Health Services Research*, 10, p. 124.

Tilley, S.A., Powick-Kumar, K.D. & Ratković, S. (2009) 'Regulatory practices and school-based research: Making sense of research ethics/review [52 paragraphs]', *Forum Qualitative Sozialforschung/Forum: Qualitative Social Research*, 10(2), Art. 32. Online journal available from http://nbn-resolving.de/urn:nbn:de:0114-fqs0902326.

Tinson, J. (2009) *Conducting research with children and adolescents.* London: Goodfellow.

Universities UK (2012) *Concordat to support research integrity.* Available for download from www.universitiesuk.ac.uk/highereducation/Documents/2012/TheConcordatToSupportResearchIntegrity.pdf.

van den Hoonaard, W.C. (ed) (2002) *Walking the tightrope: Ethical issues for qualitative researchers.* Toronto, Ontario, Canada: University of Toronto Press.

World Health Organization (2000) *Operational guidelines for ethics committees that review biomedical research.* Geneva: World Health Organization.

5 The role of the stakeholder in applied research: Managing expectations and relationships

Nóirín Hayes, Siobhán Keegan, Grainne Hickey and Gráinne Smith

Introduction

The central context for this chapter is the relatively recent but growing emphasis in both policy and practice on comprehensive community-based prevention and early intervention programmes for tackling disadvantage and developmental inequality (Sridharana et al., 2007). Initiatives such as Sure Start, Head Start and Early Head Start have now become established area-based strategies for improving outcomes and services for children and their families, as well as their communities. Building on points raised in Chapter 2, this chapter will critically examine some of the important issues underpinning collaborative approaches to research. This will incorporate three key perspectives: (1) the funder/service provider (e.g. different types of funder/service providers, including government agencies, and their differing and often diverse 'needs'); (2) the researcher(s) (e.g. the agendas and interests of the researcher(s)); (3) the community, in this instance this refers to service providers and users who are the subject of the research (e.g. how to foster 'ownership' of the research amongst participants while managing the expectations of the many diverse audiences in terms of their experiences, views of, and responses to, research). The chapter explores and describes the inter-relationships between and amongst each of these key players/sectors, while also discussing their implications. It will attempt to identify and analyse possible solutions based on the authors' collective experience of conducting applied community-based research with a range of client groups, including children and young people.

Managing expectations and relationships

Considerable progress has been made in recent years in identifying evidence-based programmes and practices which can help to reduce the likelihood of maladaptive lifepath outcomes for at-risk children (Novins et al., 2013). However, there has also been growing concern over the gap between evidence-based programmes as they are developed and the form in which they are implemented in community-based settings (Bohr et al., 2010). It is increasingly recognized that new services and supports, evidence-based or otherwise, cannot be simply transported into community-based systems and services. Indeed, there may be deeply entrenched policies, practices and processes, as well as attitudes, cultures and relationships within communities that can influence service adoption, delivery and implementation, as well as outcomes for children and families (Shapiro, Prinz & Sanders, 2012; Szapocznika et al., 2015). Pragmatic, community-based research and evaluation of community change initiatives (CCIs) (Canavan et al., 2014) can help to address the gap between theory and practice and provide important information regarding not just effectiveness, but also how and when new programmes and practices can be effectively embedded within community-based child and family services. Chapter 6 in this text considers some of the specific research design challenges and solutions in this context, while later Chapter 8 specifically reflects on evaluation of CCIs.

However, applied community-based research is a challenging undertaking and involves the successful management – by the researcher(s) and commissioners – of the wide array of relationships, multiple perspectives and expectations that arise when tendering for, planning, designing, conducting and disseminating research. This is particularly the case in large-scale projects involving numerous stakeholders, all of whom, to a greater or lesser extent, play a critical role in the successful initiation and completion of the research, in disseminating the findings and in helping to translate findings into policy and practice. Thus, it is important for applied researchers and those working with them to devote considerable energy and resources to promoting, nurturing and maintaining positive relationships at all levels, while also managing often conflicting expectations, in order to develop a shared understanding of common goals amongst all stakeholders.

The funder/commissioner perspective

Comprehensive CCIs are typically aimed at developing and implementing evidence-based and evidence-informed programmes and practices within mainstream care settings to enhance outcomes for children and their families, to encourage innovation, systems change and interagency collaboration and to build capacity with the community and across usual service systems and structures. This work frequently involves the auditing, monitoring and tracking of service implementation, delivery and outcomes through applied research and evaluation. This section will draw on the experience of a comprehensive CCI in Ireland which designed and delivered a variety of programmes for children and families in an area of disadvantage. The Tallaght West Childhood Development Initiative (CDI) is funded under the Irish government's Area-Based Childhood (ABC) Programme, which builds on the learning to date from the Prevention and Early Intervention Programme (PEIP). CDI was initially established through a partnership between the Department of Children and Youth Affairs (DCYA) and The Atlantic Philanthropies

(AP). From 2007 to 2012, CDI designed and delivered seven evidence-based and evidence-informed programmes, all of which were subject to a rigorous and complex evaluation process; it also published a number of evaluation reports, including a process evaluation of the CDI initiative as a whole (CDI, 2014 on www.twcdi.ie). It is worth noting that Chapter 8 of this text considers the case of another urban-based CCI, however in this instance from the perspective of the researchers commissioned to complete it.

Funding, commissioning and establishing a comprehensive applied research strategy involves many challenges, including ensuring that there is clarity around the roles and responsibilities of key stakeholders, as well as generating buy-in for research activities and processes. Quite often funders are also service providers who may, in some instances, have little prior experience of working with researchers and/or commissioning or managing a comprehensive research strategy. Capacity and expertise development may be needed in order to ensure that the challenges involved in applied research can be met and that the proposed research project is of a rigorous and robust nature (Minkler & Wallerstein, 2010). In this situation, CDI was a commissioner of research and programmes; funding was granted from outside sources and programme design and delivery was the responsibility of the CDI. However, CDI did not directly deliver programmes, but instead commissioned local services and agencies to deliver the programmes. In acting as a conduit between the funders, researchers and the community CDI provided a coordinating locus with the potential to allow for flexibility, understanding and good communication. In acting as a fulcrum, CDI worked to provide clarity around the respective roles and responsibilities of key stakeholders, as well as highlighting pathways through which research activities could be implemented in an efficient and ethical manner, with a view to ensuring that research could meet community/organizational needs. Some examples of the resources and activities put in place by CDI in order to meet the challenges of a multifaceted applied research strategy and facilitate it are described below.

In working with each stakeholder group, CDI identified relevant needs crucial to undertaking the research. Structures were put in place to ensure transparency, clarity and support with the design and participation in the research. The structures included an 'Expert Advisory Committee' (EAC), which offered an opportunity to validate and tease through the complexities of the proposed research, and an Implementation Support Group (ISG) to consider the detail of the programmes and ensure that they remained true to the strategic objectives and met identified needs. This group was made up of local lead agencies, including schools and statutory and non-statutory agencies. These groups reported to the CDI Board, which included representatives from the community to ensure that the voice of the community was heard and that the language used by CDI and the research teams was accessible to the community.

Taking account of research findings on the importance of communication in community-based research (Novins et al., 2013; Canavan et al., 2014;

Herbert et al., 2009), CDI developed a specific staff team comprising operational staff (Quality Specialists) and a Research and Evaluation Officer (REO) to enhance communication links across various stakeholders. Having members on the staff team whose sole responsibility was to liaise between the research teams, the EAC and operational staff ensured consistency as well as effective communication. This also allowed the operational staff to concentrate on programme design and delivery. The REO met with the evaluation teams every month until the programmes and research methodology were bedded down. Thereafter, meetings were held on a quarterly basis, with close communication maintained via emails and phone calls. In addition to this, all research teams met as a group twice a year to discuss the research and cross-cutting themes. The REO role was vital in ensuring that the complex research studies ran as smoothly and effectively as possible. Coordinating data collection timelines in order to minimize research burden in the community was central to this.

Given the complexities and variance of the research undertaken, it is important to be clear about stakeholders' needs. Close working relationships, collaboration and open communication are key to ensuring needs are heard and addressed (Jones, 2008; Nutley, Walter and Davies, 2007; McIlrath et al., 2014). CDI's strategic plan and funding allocation were based on three years of consultation. When the organization moved from the planning to implementation phase (Burke, Morris and McGarrigle, 2012), further consultations were held in order to ensure the buy-in and continued engagement of all stakeholders. Clarity in communication is a central requirement for community-based research, particularly finding a common language which allows all stakeholders to feel empowered (Herbert et al., 2009). Understanding the 'language' of research took time, both for CDI as purveyors and for the commissioned services.

A recurring theme throughout the research project for both service providers and CDI as funders was finding an acceptable balance between evidence-based or needs-led initiatives. Was one informing the other? And, most importantly, where did CDI want to be? Could the two be divided and should goals or approach be changed to fit in with the research? Careful thought needed to be given to this at the research design stage. When considering the research methodology the funders had to ensure that it would 'fit' with service delivery. Awareness and articulation of potential challenges allowed the process to be managed with effective consultation and collaboration at the outset and with ongoing open communication. In the case of CDI's Early Years Service, consideration was given to the complexities of using a Randomized Control Trial. Discussions were held on the ethics of randomly assigning children in an early years service, and in the end a decision was made to randomly assign the services rather than the children; thus, a randomized cluster design was utilized (Hayes, Siraj-Blatchford and Keegan, 2013). When allocating the children into control or intervention groups in our afterschool literacy programme – 'Doodle Den' – a set of twins was referred to the programme. As it happened, one twin was assigned to the control group and the other twin to the intervention group. Again, following discussions, it was decided for ethical reasons to assign both twins to the intervention groups (Biggart et al., 2012). These complexities would not have been picked up or discussed were it not for the nature and close relationships CDI had with both the schools and research teams.

Given that this level of research was new to both CDI and service providers, opportunities were created at various points to discuss concerns, direction and purpose of the research. As a strategy for managing the expectations of settings and participants, CDI arranged for the lead researchers to meet with the frontline staff and parents to identify, discuss and resolve any issues that were of concern. Developing these close relationships and maintaining them throughout the research period was crucial and should be factored in when considering using applied research.

Being a commissioner of programmes and research necessitates good working relationships, reflecting the collaborative and responsive approach to research considered in Chapter 2. This was key to the successful undertaking of the varied and complex research projects. Regular meetings were held between operational staff and the service providers, where issues were discussed and clarified. These meetings and issues were fed back to the REO, who could liaise directly with the researchers and EAC as required. In addition, training was provided to fieldworkers to ensure a collaborative approach to the research. Being part of research as opposed to having it 'done to' you allows for achieving better buy-in, engagement and collaboration (Farrell & Weitman, 2007).

While ensuring a rigorous collaborative approach to the research is important, so too is the dissemination of the findings and feedback loops. CDI gave this careful consideration and decided to hold reflection groups, round tables and launches once the research teams had reported. The purpose of the reflection groups was to give those who were involved in the research an opportunity to hear from the researchers what the evaluation found and a chance to discuss the implications of the findings. These reflection groups were held locally, with services providers, parents and other relevant local agencies attending. This local dimension, often a challenge to researchers, is key to community-based research and affects not only "the choice of research focus but also the research methods used, the process of learning from the research, and its impact" (ICPHR, 2013, p. 9).

Reports that had major statistically significant findings were launched by the relevant government minister to a wider audience, with press releases issued. This helped to validate the work of the service providers and the programmes they had being delivering. Round tables were also hosted and attended by relevant senior policymakers and influencers in order to reflect upon the findings and to consider the implications and possibilities for replication. Not all research findings were positive, and some research reported no programme effect. Managing such findings was important to the overall prevention and early intervention initiatives and, while disappointing to some stakeholders, this does provide valuable learning for the commissioners and researchers (Finklestein and Fishbach, 2012). As well as publishing the reports, policy briefs were developed which took the learnings and recommendations from the reports in order to inform policy and practice. Conferences and seminars were held with a variety of audiences to share these policy recommendations.

When commissioning applied research, it is important that all those involved have an initial and on-going opportunity to discuss and understand the purpose of the research and the impacts it will have on practice. Collaboration is vital to ensure a smooth undertaking of applied research in practice settings and to allow for the research findings to have practical relevance for on-going service delivery and development. Key elements contributing to successful community-based research include: clear governance structures which can leverage capacity and expertise; open and transparent communication channels; a designated person to liaise with the research teams; an operational staff to enable efficient research activities; and processes which can meet the identified and agreed upon needs of all key stakeholders.

The researcher perspective

With growing emphasis on evidence-based services for children and families there has been, in line with international trends, a concomitant increase in investment in research. This has paralleled a trend in both international and Irish policy towards the expansion of area-based prevention and early intervention programmes which focus on providing parenting supports and which target childhood inequality. There is now a recognized need for further experimental and quasi-experimental trials, implementation research and cost-effectiveness studies which are conducted in applied community-based settings and which can inform service development and implementation and policy in relation to child and family provisions (Allen, 2011). However, conducting research in applied community-based settings is a challenging undertaking for the researcher.

Recent significant advances in the delivery and testing of prevention and early intervention programmes provide an expanding evidence base for 'what works' for parents and children (Axford et al., 2012; Webster-Stratton & Taylor, 2001). Despite this progress, there remain pressing questions regarding the optimal content, timing, intensity and length of community-based services and interventions (Bakerman-Kranenburg, van IJzendoorn & Juffer, 2003; Buchanan, Miller & Wallerstein, 2007; Szapocznika et al., 2015). Furthermore, prevention and early intervention programmes such as CDI are often multifaceted in nature and their success and/or failure often depend on the context in which they are implemented, while traditional research methods, including controlled trials, provide little insight into how such interventions work or which components of complex interventions and contextual factors contribute to outcomes (Oakley et al., 2006). Thus, many questions regarding the conditions, processes or programme components that influence the effectiveness of child- and family-focused interventions remain unanswered. Addressing these questions through applied community-based research is an important undertaking. However, evaluating complex CCIs is challenging for a wide variety of reasons, ranging from the interpersonal to the methodological.

Researchers and community-based stakeholders can come to the research with distinct 'world views'. Applied research can be complicated by conflicting values and expectations between researchers and community-based stakeholders in the research process. Researchers' values and agendas can be distinctly different from those of community-based service providers and community members with regard to research design and methodology. Indeed, researchers may encounter resistance to research implementation at a community level (McIlrath et al., 2014). Researchers set out to explore the effectiveness of community-based interventions and services, often using randomized controlled trials as the 'gold standard' for research evidence. More and more, experimental methods are being used to conduct evaluations in applied service settings, yet researchers may be faced with discomfort and/or ethical objections around the idea of randomization in community-based settings and social intervention (Buchanan et al., 2007). There can be concerns about the ethics of withholding a potentially effective intervention from community members, particularly those who are vulnerable, 'harder to reach' and/or have complex needs. The main reason for conducting rigorous evaluations of community-based services is to create evidence from which the community can benefit, and researchers, like practitioners, are interested in addressing social, health or mental health inequalities and informing the development of high-quality services and interventions for communities. However, conflicts may stem from a lack of experience with research processes and a lack of joint understanding around the aims and usefulness of the research. Fears regarding stigmatization of community members as problematic or dysfunctional and/or concerns over the implications of research design for service delivery and service funding may also give rise to research resistance (Durham Community Research Team, 2011). While research can play a vital role in producing valid findings which practitioners and policymakers can rely on to inform service development and delivery, there is a need to articulate clearly the reasons why research is conducted and what it can offer the community. This can help to address any assumptions or opinions that may exist regarding researchers' roles and the utility of research, and provide a foundation for positive relationships between researchers and the community with whom they will be conducting the research.

Hayes, Ilan and Kelly (2008) found that there can be a wide gulf in perceptions and expectations between professional agents and residents of disadvantaged communities caused by complex social, economic and cultural factors, a finding mirrored in a number of the CDI programmes. Community trust can support optimal participant recruitment, engagement and retention (Minkler, 2005). Failure to engage and retain parents, for instance, may have a deleterious effect on the quality of community-based research and may undermine the overarching utility of the findings. Dialogue is an important step towards mutual appreciation and collaborative action. Researchers need to listen to and learn about the community that they are researching (Finkelstein and Fishbach, 2012). They also need to be aware of power differentials in order for community-based research to be implemented effectively and satisfactorily for all stakeholders involved in the process. The traditional research process where the researchers define the problem and research questions, develop the study design, implement data collection procedures, carry out analysis and finalize report writing and data dissemination is often not applicable to community-based evaluations of complex interventions (Michener et al., 2012). Indeed

> Consistent with constructivist and critical theory paradigms and their emphasis on the socially created nature of scientific knowledge, a fundamental characteristic of community-based research … is the emphasis on the participation and influence of nonacademic researchers in the process of creating knowledge.
>
> (Israel et al., 1998, p. 177)

Community-based research therefore necessitates a different approach to more traditional research processes and incorporates partnership building and collaborative development of research aims and objectives, joint recruitment of research participants, data collection, analysis and the dissemination of findings into the research programme.

Building good working relationships with stakeholders involved in developing and implementing interventions is challenging in the context of community-based research, particularly when the researchers finds themselves in a situation where they are being remunerated by the person, group or organization that they are also evaluating. Indeed, important issues of 'turf', ownership and responsibilities can ensue. Research and evaluation can be seen as threatening to stakeholders who hold vested interests in portraying an intervention/service in a positive light. On the other hand, collaborative processes can be seen as a threat to researchers' objectivity, choices of methodology and research activities and ownership of the research. Nevertheless, achieving high quality applied research requires positive relationships with stakeholders. Without such a foundation, close observation and analysis of the intervention can be difficult (Moore et al., 2015). The traditional research 'rules' of 'objectivity' and 'rigour' may initially jar with the concept of joint participation and collaboration in research development and implementation. Importantly, it is not that the researcher values of objectivity and evaluation rigour cannot be upheld; nor does it preclude the use of experimental methods. However, the processes by which they are pursued may differ, while it is also important that such imperatives are balanced with the need for relevance for community members and the larger goals of community-based stakeholders (Potter, 2006). In a review of community-based research, Jagosh et al. (2015) reported that developing and strengthening partnerships across stakeholders was best built on trust. To achieve such trust, there must be continued commitment to power sharing and systems for co-governance. They found that secure and well-established trust-related mechanisms at three levels – context, mechanism and outcome – yielded greater sustainability and transformation of effective programmes. Cooke and Kothari (2001) describe the pitfalls of three 'tyrannies' when it comes to community-based, participatory research, challenging researchers to avoid them. They are: the tyranny of decision making, whereby community decisions are overridden by experts; the tyranny of the group, where those in power in communities retain and reinforce their agenda simply due to their being the loudest and therefore the easiest to hear; and the tyranny of methods, where, in an attempt to be inclusive and accessible for the community, research methods are used that may not challenge the status quo within that community. Thus, the researcher or research team must be aware of and sensitive to communities' values and priorities when conducting research in community settings, while also maintaining sufficient independence to critically observe and analyse the process and practice of intervention, as well as the outcomes for the communities which are served (Moore et al., 2015). It is also important to follow community implementation schedules in order to allow stakeholders to engage in the research in balance with their community commitments (Jones & Wells, 2007). After all, the primary goal of applied research is typically to find out how the community may benefit, be it from the research process itself or from services or other community efforts.

Overall, researchers themselves may benefit greatly from building positive working relationships with stakeholders. Working collaboratively with community stakeholders can augment planning processes by bringing to light contextual factors that need to be accounted for in the design of the study and in helping to identify potential problems, needs and barriers to research implementation alongside potential solutions and viable research strategies (Bieluch et al., 2016; Newman et al., 2011). This additional dimension can be captured through including a process evaluation as part of the overall research design. Thus, building strong evidence of what works for children and families increasingly involves mixed-methodological research studies which address not just questions of effectiveness, but also the 'how' and 'why' of programme efficacy (Munro & Bloor, 2010). Indeed, there are many instances where traditional/gold standard research methods of randomization may not be feasible, and there are also limits to the insights that outcome evaluations can offer. Multimodal research, combining outcome-focused and process-oriented research methods, can help to establish an evidence base for effective practices, processes, services and supports, while also furnishing decision makers and service providers with important information regarding how and when prevention and early programmes may be effectively embedded within community-based child and family usual care services (Moore et al., 2015). Importantly, researchers themselves, and not just community partners, may also be on a significant learning curve when it comes to the multifaceted, dynamic and methodologically challenging nature of applied research processes. Therefore, it is important for researchers to be open and honest about their own constraints, limitations and knowledge gaps in order to build authentic partnerships and engender collaborative working practices between researchers and a range of community-based stakeholders.

Data ownership and the dissemination of findings can also be an area of conflict in community-based research. One of the key ambitions of researchers is to publish in academic journals; however, such publications often do not make an impact at a community or policy level. Working with community stakeholders can help to target messages towards key decision makers and improve the impact of the research (Michener et al., 2012). There may also be concerns amongst community stakeholders when research findings do not support the effectiveness of the programme or may be less positive than anticipated. This is particularly the case where it is perceived that future service delivery and funding will be threatened. However, ineffective strategies can continue to be implemented if negative or non-supportive findings are not published (Nutley et al., 2008). Conversely, evidence-based practices may not be widely adopted, even when strong evidence for effectiveness and cost-effectiveness exists. Researchers and evaluators, therefore, need to assist service providers, policymakers and other decision makers to appreciate the boundaries and limitations of research if they are to learn from research and improve the quality of service delivery at a community level in an informed way. The findings from research programmes need to be made available in a format that is accessible and useable for community partners and policymakers. Seeking stakeholder input into communication plans and dissemination strategies can help to mitigate these risks and ultimately help all stakeholders to benefit from the research.

Undertaking community-based and applied research can be mutually beneficial for researchers, participants, service providers and policymakers. However, research in applied settings can be beset by conflicting agendas and disagreements. Communication, cooperation and trust are fundamental to resolving these issues and ensuring that a high quality research process can be put in place and maintained (Jones & Wells, 2007; Jagosh et al., 2015). At its best, research can help to build community knowledge and inform evidence-based practice. Furthermore, the knowledge, skills and expertise of the researcher can be enhanced through engagement and cooperation with community stakeholders. Indeed, working collaboratively can help to enrich and improve the quality of community-based research through careful and collaborative development of research programmes that capture and address issues which are of concern at a community level and can influence service development and delivery, as well as ultimately having beneficial outcomes for recruitment of participants and the dissemination of findings.

The community stakeholder perspective

Despite improvements in ethical oversight (as discussed in Chapter 4), communities and participants may nonetheless be taken advantage of to a greater or lesser extent by researchers who feel the imperative to collect data at all costs (Tinson, 2009). There is limited literature on the involvement of communities and community-based stakeholders in the design and execution of applied community-based research (Axford et al., 2012). However, it is increasingly recognized that such involvement may be vital to overcoming common barriers to recruiting and engaging stakeholders with both interventions and research studies (Davis, McDonald & Axford, 2012).

Deloria (1992) coined the terms 'helicopter research' (for geographically remote communities) and 'drive-by research' (for urban communities) to characterize the phenomenon of researchers arriving for fleeting visits to take the information they needed and leaving nothing in return. Many communities taken advantage of in the past by researchers are now demanding rights in relation to research participation and a say in who does the research and how it is done (DeBruyn et al., 2001; Wallerstein & Duran, 2008). Lasker and Weiss (2003) point out that the often complex questions being researched in community settings cannot be solved by any group, sector or person working alone. Moreover, for researchers to fully understand and compose the correct research questions, it is important for research participants (or at least those from the target population) to become involved in the research at the research planning and commissioning stage (McIlrath et al., 2014). This fulfils at least two of the principles of community-based research as suggested by Israel et al. (1998) – building on strengths and resources in the community, and facilitating a co-learning and empowering process that attends to issues such as social inequalities.

Duran and Duran (1999) recommend placing funding and decision-making with the communities' lead agencies and then subcontracting to researchers. One way to promote meaningful participation is for researchers to take on board and actively seek the knowledge of community members and research participants before, during and after the research process (Bishop, 1994; Labonte, 1994; Yeich & Levine, 1992). It is not enough to pay lip service to community participation by having focus groups with participants at the beginning and end of the research; rather, community representatives should have a more active and on-going role in the research. Wallerstein and Duran (2008) advocate involving community members in the decision-making process at each step, from research commissioning to data collection, analysis and interpretation. It is important for researchers to examine intricate sub-relationships within communities when seeking participant involvement, however. Participants should be truly representative of their communities

(Green & Mercer, 2001; Jewkes & Murcott, 1998) rather than simply a representation of the most powerful level within the community (Durham Community Research Team, 2011). Participation in research by members of a community may include acting as a joint grant holder on a given research initiative, helping to identify research priorities, providing expert advice and support for research activities, providing feedback and support on the development of information leaflets and research promotional materials and assisting and participating with research activities (Hayes, Buckland & Tarpey, 2012).

Building on community strengths and resources allows for a strengthening of the overall research through tapping in to a base of social capital within the community, which may be used to inform the development of community-relevant research questions as well as to garner participants and fieldworkers, access hard-to-reach participants and eventually implement changes. Studies have found that peer education, whereby HIV clinical trial participants became educators for new recruits to the programme, increased the retention rate and led to better engagement by the target population in spite of cultural differences between participants and the research team (Naidoo, Morar & Ramjee, 2013). Wallerstein and Duran (2008) sum up the complexity well by saying of participation in research that:

> Participation should not be seen as a magic bullet but as a complex and iterative process, which can change, grow or diminish, based on the unfolding of power relations and the historical and social context of the research project.
>
> (p. 32)

They recommend that self-reflexivity in researchers and with the community participants can help to guard against such "tyrannies" and "can inspire a continual cycle of learning" (p. 32) about what works and what does not work in research. Due recognition and publication of such successes and failures can help inform prospective research studies, researchers and participants.

Conclusion

The fact that the term for describing research participants has moved from the subjective to the participative is perhaps telling of the changing face of research participation in recent years. There is increased recognition that local community knowledge increases our understanding of the complex interactions among economic, social and behavioural factors that contribute to disparities, and that these should therefore inform the design of interventions aimed at reducing these disparities (Hayes et al., 2008; Hayes et al., 2013). Community-based research provides a voice and a role to individuals within communities, while also attempting to atone for the historical tendency of researchers to 'subject' community members to research. Addressing these issues draws on many of the principles, discussed in Chapter 2. The principle of co-learning and empowerment is particularly important when conducting research in community settings and can be the key to the success of community interventions. The advantages of engaging community participants meaningfully in research is that the research which is generated is culturally relevant and more readily translatable into action through programmes or interventions (Jacquez, Vaughn & Wagner, 2013).

Researchers must acknowledge that there may be inequalities between themselves and community participants, which may shape how, or if, they participate in the research process. Research participants may have different reasons for participating in the research than the researchers intend, such as employment, empowerment, desire to express needs/difficulties and capacity building. If done properly, the research process can answer research questions that concern the community as well as having the added advantage of empowering individuals within communities to have more power over their lives and over what happens to benefit their community.

References

Allen, G. (2011) *Early intervention: The next steps. An independent report to her majesty's government*. London: Cabinet Office.

Axford, N. *et al.* (2012) 'Engaging parents in parenting programs: Lessons from research and practice', *Children and Youth Services Review*, 34, pp. 2061–2071.

Bakerman-Kranenburg, M.J., van IJzendoorn, M.H. & Juffer, H. (2003) 'Less is more: Meta-analysis of sensitivity and attachment intervention in early childhood', *Psychological Bulletin*, 129, pp. 195–215.

Bieluch, K.H. et al. (2016) 'Transdisciplinary research partnerships in sustainability science: an examination of stakeholder participation preferences', *Sustainability Science*, first online: 21 March 2016, pp. 1–18.

Biggart, A. *et al.* (2012) *Evaluation of the effectiveness of the Childhood Development's Doodle Den Literacy Programme*. Dublin: Child Development Initiative.

Bishop, R. (1994) 'Initiating empowering research?' *New Zealand Journal of Educational Studies*, 29, pp. 175–188.

Bohr, Y. *et al.* (2010) 'Community-based parenting training: Do adapted evidence-based programmes improve parent–infant interactions?' *Journal of Reproductive and Infant Psychology*, 28, pp. 55–68.

Buchanan, D.R., Miller, F.G. & Wallerstein, N. (2007) 'Ethical issues in community-based participatory research: Balancing rigorous research with community participation in community intervention studies', *Progress in Community Health Partnerships: Research, Education, and Action*, 1, pp. 153–160.

Burke, K., Morris, K. and McGarrigle, L. (2012) *An introductory guide to implementation: Terms, concepts and frameworks*. Dublin: Centre for Effective Services. Available from www.effectiveservices.org/images/uploads/file/Guide%20to%20implementation%20concepts%20and%20frameworks%20Final%20for%20web.pdf.

Canavan, J. *et al.* (2014) *Leading community change: Delivering better outcomes in an Irish community. Childhood development initiative final process evaluation report*. Dublin: Childhood Development Initiative.

Cooke, B. & Kothari, U. (eds) (2001) *Participation: The new tyranny?* London: Zed Books.

Davis, F.A., McDonald, L. & Axford, N. (2012) 'Technique is not enough: A framework for ensuring that evidence-based parenting programmes are socially inclusive'. Discussion paper. British Psychological Society. Available from www.bps.org.uk/system/files/images/tine.pdf (Accessed 29 February 2016).

DeBruyn, L. *et al.* (2001) 'Child maltreatment in American Indian and Alaska Native communities: Integrating culture, history, and public health for intervention and prevention', *Child Maltreatment*, 6(2), pp. 89–102.

Deloria, V. (1992) 'Indians, archaeologists, and the future', *American Antiquity*, 57, pp. 595–598.

Duran, E. & Duran, B. (1995) *Native-American postcolonial psychology.* Albany: State University of New York Press.

Durham Community Research Team (2011) *Community based participatory research: Ethical challenges.* Durham: Centre for Social Justice and Community Action.

Farrell, J.B. and Weitman, C.J. (2007) 'Action research fosters empowerment and learning communities', *The Delta Kappa Gamma Bulletin*, 73(3), pp. 36–40.

Finkelstein, S.R. and Fishbach, A. (2012) 'Tell me what I did wrong: Experts seek and respond to negative feedback', *Journal of Consumer Research*, 0093–5301/2012/3901–0003. doi:10.1086/661934

Green, L.W. & Mercer, S.L. (2001) 'Can public health researchers and agencies reconcile the push from funding bodies and the pull from communities?' *American Journal of Public Health*, 91(12), pp. 1926–1929.

Hayes, H., Buckland, S. & Tarpey, M. (2012) 'Briefing notes for researchers: Public involvement in NHS, public health and social care research', *INVOLVE*. Available from www.involve.nihr.ac.uk/resource-centre/resource-for-researchers (Accessed 29 February 2016).

Hayes, N., Ilan, J. & Kelly, S. (2008) *Our opinions matter: An action research project with parents and children in the canal communities: Final report.* Dublin: Canal Communities Partnership.

Hayes, N., Siraj-Blatchford, I. and Keegan, S. (2013) *Evaluation of the Early Years Programme of the Childhood Development Initiative.* Dublin: Child Development Initiative.

Hebert, J.R. *et al.* (2009) 'Interdisciplinary, Translational and Community-Based Participatory Research: Finding a Common Language to Improve Cancer Research', *Cancer Epidemiology, Biomarkers and Prevention*, 18(4), pp. 1213–1217.

ICPHR (International Collaboration for Participatory Health Research) (2013) *Position paper 1: What is participatory health research?* Berlin: International Collaboration for Participatory Health Research.

Israel, B.A. *et al.* (1998) 'Review of community-based research: Assessing partnership approaches to improve public health', *Annual Review of Public Health*, 19, pp. 173–202.

Jacquez, F., Vaughn, L.M. & Wagner, E. (2013) 'Youth as partners, participants or passive recipients: A review of children and adolescents in community-based participatory research (CBPR)', *American Journal of Community Psychology*, 51(1–2), pp. 176–189.

Jagosh, J. *et al.* (2015) 'A realist evaluation of community-based participatory research: Partnership synergy, trust building and related ripple effects', *BMC Public Health*. doi:10.1186/s12889–015–1949–1

Jewkes, R. & Murcott, A. (1998) 'Community representatives: Representing the "community"?', *Social Science & Medicine*, 46(7), pp. 843–858.

Jones, P. (2008) *Communicating strategy*. Hampshire, UK: Gower.

Jones, L. & Wells, K. (2007) 'Strategies for academic and clinician engagement in community–participatory partnered research', *Journal of the American Medical Association*, 297, pp. 407–410.

Labonte, R. (1994) 'Health promotion and empowerment: Reflections on professional practice', *Health Education Quarterly*, 21, pp. 253–268.

Lasker, R.D. & Weiss, E.S. (2003) 'Broadening participation in community problem solving: A multidisciplinary model to support collaborative practice and research', *Journal of Urban Health*, 80(1), pp. 14–47.

McIlrath, L. *et al.* (2014) 'Emerging policy and practices on community-based research – Perspectives from the island of Ireland', in Munck, R. *et al.* (eds) *Higher education and community-based research: Creating a global vision*. New York, NY: Palgrave Macmillan.

Michener, L. *et al.* (2012) 'Aligning the goals of community-engaged research: Why and how academic health centers can successfully engage with communities to improve health', *Academic Medicine*, 87, pp. 285–291.

Milgram, S. (1963) 'Behavioral study of obedience', *The Journal of Abnormal and Social Psychology*, 67(4), p. 371.

Minkler, M. (2005) 'Community-based research partnerships: Challenges and opportunities', *Journal of Urban Health*, 82, pp. ii3-ii12.

Minkler, M. & Wallerstein, N. (eds) (2010) *Community-based participatory research for health: From process to outcomes*. San Francisco, CA: John Wiley & Sons.

Moore, G. F., Audrey, S., Barker, M., Bond, L., Bonell, C., Hardeman, W., Moore, L., O'Cathain, A., Tinati, T., Wight, D. & Baird, J. (2015) 'Process evaluation of complex interventions: Medical Research Council guidance', *British Medical Journal*, 350, p. h1258.

Munro, A. & Bloor, M. (2010) 'Process evaluation: The new miracle ingredient in public health research?' *Qualitative Research*, 10, pp. 699–713.

Naidoo, S., Morar, N.S. & Ramjee, G. (2013) 'Participants as community-based peer educators: Impact on a clinical trial site in KwaZulu-Natal', *South African Journal of Science*, 109(7–8), pp. 1–5.

NewmanS.D. *et al.* (2011) 'Community advisory boards in community-based participatory research: A synthesis of best processes', *Preventing Chronic Disease: Public Health Research, Practice, and Policy*, 8(3), p. A70.

Novins, D.K. *et al.* (2013) 'Dissemination and implementation of evidence-based practices for child and adolescent mental health: a systematic review', *Journal of the American Academy of Child and Adolescent Psychiatry*, 52, pp. 1009–1025.

Nutley, S., Walter, I. and Davies, H. (2007) *Using evidence: How research can inform public services*. Bristol: Policy Press.

Oakley, A. *et al.* (2006) 'Process evaluation in randomised controlled trials of complex interventions', *British Medical Journal*, 332, pp. 413–416.

Potter, C. (2006) 'Programme evaluation', in Terre Blanche, M., Durrheim, K. & Painter, D. (eds) *Research in practice: Applied methods for the social sciences*. 2nd edn. Cape Town: UCT Press, pp. 409–428.

Shapiro, C.J., Prinz, R.J. & Sanders, M.R. (2012) 'Facilitators and barriers to implementation of an evidence-based parenting intervention to prevent child maltreatment: The Triple P-Positive Parenting Program', *Child Maltreatment*, 17, pp. 86–95.

Sridharana, S. *et al.* (2007) 'Analysis of strategic plans to assess planning for sustainability of comprehensive community initiatives', *Evaluation and Program Planning*, 30, pp. 105–113.

Szapocznika, J. *et al.* (2015) 'Brief strategic family therapy: Implementing evidence-based models in community settings', *Psychotherapy Research*, 25. doi:10.1080/10503307.2013.856044

Tinson, J. (2009) *Conducting research with children and adolescents.* Oxford, UK: Goodfellow Publishers.

Wallerstein, N. & Duran, B. (2008) 'The theoretical, historical, and practice roots of CBPR', in Minkler, M. & Wallerstein, N. (eds) *Community-based participatory research for health: From process to outcomes.* San Francisco, CA: Wiley, pp. 25–46.

Webster-Stratton, C. & Taylor, T. (2001) 'Nipping early risk factors in the bud: Preventing substance abuse, delinquency, and violence in adolescence through interventions targeted at young children (0–8 years)', *Prevention Science*, 2, pp. 165–192.

Yeich, S. & Levine, R. (1992) 'Participatory research's contribution to a conceptualization of empowerment', *Journal of Applied Social Psychology*, 22, pp. 1894–1908.

6 Developing a detailed design for research with communities

Suzanne Guerin and Catherine Comiskey

Introduction

The aim of this book is to explore the key aspects and phases involved in conducting research in community settings with children, families and other key stakeholders. Within this context, this chapter explores the challenges of designing research for these contexts. While the content of this chapter will, by its nature, be directed at readers who aim to or must design a study for successful implementation in community settings, the material will also be insightful for those commissioning research in these settings, as well as practitioners and policymakers charged with developing services in line with research.

The convention in research design involves several core features. These include a clear and valuable research question, an effective research method that is appropriate for the key question, the identification and measurement of appropriate data or variables, a defendable sampling strategy and a comprehensive data management, data analysis and dissemination plan. Conducting research in a real world community setting, however, presents several challenges to these conventions. This chapter considers some of the challenges evident when designing research in community, health and social care settings. These challenges include agreement on the research question by a range of competing stakeholders who may vary in perspective and physical location and the possible tension between a rigorous design and the need for flexibility in implementation. In addition to these challenges, there is the need for the research and researchers to engage meaningfully from inception to impact with those who live and work within the community.

Despite these challenges, research excellence demands the adherence to international best practice, independent of the approach or framework used by the researcher. The aim of this chapter is to discuss and elucidate these challenges, to evaluate and propose a range of responses to these and to reflect on their implications when conducting the highest quality research in a demanding community environment. This chapter addresses in sequential order the challenges facing the researcher when designing a study in community settings.

Starting out

Starting a research project in community settings can involve different points of entry. Commissioners of research will have produced a tender document highlighting their anticipated needs and objectives, a process discussed in detail in Chapter 3. However, tenders can range from highly developed calls for a specific study to more general requests for input to a developing process. The researchers may be responding to such a tender document, submitting a grant application for additional funding or working within a community organization to develop a piece of research. Each of these will have different challenges, but the core issues are the same. The first is identifying the focus of the project and agreeing clear research questions that will guide the research.

Identifying and clarifying the key question

One of the first tasks for the researcher is identifying the key question from a request for tender document, expression of interest or similar document. For a tender to be successful, the researcher must make the first attempt at identifying and clarifying the key question from a document that may have been written by many stakeholders with varying views, agendas, expectations and needs, and perhaps with varying levels of expertise in research methods. In real world or community-based research the varying stakeholders may not have contributed equally both professionally and financially to the project. It can be helpful where there has been time and support for the tendering organization to secure research support in developing the document. Nevertheless, the researcher must be able to reflect the tender from the perspective of all stakeholders and endeavour to identify from the documentation the key question of greatest value and benefit to all involved. Depending on the nature of the call, this may be a negotiated or a collaborative process between the commissioner and the research team, which may be done through a tender question and response process or a more interactive engagement with research partners.

The key research question is one of the cornerstones of the research, and many additional questions will be added and developed to help answer the key question. Regardless of the research design chosen, the overarching aim or hypothesis of the study will be based on the key question. Additional questions and hypotheses will follow within the study, and these combined contribute towards building up the evidence that will provide the final answer. This highlights the need for all parties to be happy with the research question. With this in mind, simplicity is the core value or kernel of the key question. For example, 'Does the treatment work?', 'Is the intervention effective?', 'What is the scale of the problem?' and 'Where must cutbacks or developments be made?' are all examples of strong, clear key questions that require strong, clear answers.

To highlight the way in which a strong key question will lead to further research questions, let us take one question – 'Is the intervention effective?'– as an example: Even an apparently simple question such as this may need to be broken down further into its component parts. In this example, it must be decided at what level the outcome of the intervention is to be measured. Is it required that effects are obtained at the level of the individual, the community or the wider society, or all three? Is one level of greater priority than another? In school-based intervention research the parent stakeholder may wish to see change at the individual level, the principal at the school level and the funder of the research at the societal or policy level. These three levels give rise to further questions, such as, 'Is the intervention effective for the pupil, the school and society?' The single outcome of impact or change must also be clarified. An outcome in a school-based intervention may be an improved reading ability at the individual level, decreased absenteeism at a school level and increased community engagement at a society level. This diverse range of outcomes adds to the body of questions that contribute to and support the overall key question. This issue is further illustrated in relation to substance misuse research in Box 6.1.

Box 6.1 Reflecting on research questions in substance misuse research

A further example of how the key question can be both simple and yet very broad is evident in community substance misuse treatment research. The need for the evaluation of treatment for substance misuse at national and community level has been recognized across the globe from the United States (Hubbard, Craddock & Anderson, 2003) to Europe (UK – Jones et al., 2009; Ireland – Comiskey et al., 2009) to Australia (Teesson et al., 2006).

The simple research question – 'Is treatment effective?' – has been addressed internationally, yet it will have varied meaning for different services with differing philosophies and differing target groups. A network of local community support centres with a harm reduction philosophy may consider treatment effective if the level of risk to the individual and their family is reduced. A national medical centre with an abstinence philosophy may consider treatment effective if treatment leads to the cessation of substance misuse and a government agency may consider treatment effective if levels of crime in the community are reduced.

Clearly, while the overarching key question on whether on or not treatment is effective is applicable to all interest groups, each group will interpret the meaning of the question in a different manner, and within any tender, grant or funding proposal the researcher must present the key question in such a way that it may be both universally applicable and simple, yet is capable of the depth and breadth required to be meaningful and useful to a range of stakeholders.

A further challenge to the researcher is the need to devise a research question that can be flexible and adaptable during the research. This is particularly important in longitudinal research where the research question must be capable of responding to external factors that may influence the research in both a negative and positive way. Colin Robson, in his excellent text Real World Research (2011), refers to fixed and flexible research designs, recognizing the adaptations that may be needed as the research is implemented. This flexibility may be in the best interests of the commissioner and other stakeholders also, whose own organizational needs might change during the longitudinal research process. Building upon the substance misuse case above, if the key question is treatment impact, then the researcher may need to refine this if resources change. For example, if recruitment is slow, the follow-up period for a second interview may need to be extended. Alternatively, if the resources allow, the key question may change. If, at the first follow-up point, for example, analysis reveals that indeed treatment works, then the key question may change to, 'Are treatment effects sustainable?' In this example, the possibility of adapting the question is of value to the funding organization and a discussion between the parties regarding possible revisions to the question at the heart of the research may be beneficial to all involved.

Research design in an applied context

Once the question has been identified, the next step is the design of the study that will address that question. As Robson (2011) says, "[research] design is concerned with turning research questions into projects" (p. 79). However, the process of design is not a simple one, even at the best of times. In terms of research design, research conducted in real world or applied settings can draw from across disciplinary preferences and, thus, the options open to research teams are many and varied. For example, a research team that includes both researchers with a background in psychology and those with a background in sociology can draw on techniques ranging from experimental studies to inductive and exploratory techniques.

In Ireland the growth of multidisciplinary research centres such as the UNESCO Child and Family Research Centre at the National University of Ireland, Galway, the Trinity Research in Childhood Centre at Trinity College Dublin and the UCD Geary Institute at University College Dublin represent a framework in which researchers from many disciplines can work together on applied projects. Internationally, there are many examples of multidisciplinary research centres, including the Thomas Coram Research Institute in London, the Yale Child Study Centre in the United States and the Heidelberg Institute of Public Health in Germany. Another benefit of these national and international multidisciplinary centres is that there is generally an agreed orientation or vision that unites the members of the team and underlies the work of the centre. There can be no doubt that the variety that comes from research teams, and particularly multidisciplinary groups, allows researchers the scope to tailor the design of a project to the intricacies of the research question, the setting and the stakeholders, who ultimately benefit from this expertise. For example, a study commissioned for the national arm of an international organization would benefit from a design that can be applied internationally.

Another reason why this variation in approach is important is that research design in real world community settings does not map neatly onto the conventions of traditional research design, which are often dominated by discussions of quantitative and qualitative components. Rather than considering these positions as representing opposite philosophies, it is more useful to imagine these options as consisting of a continuum which includes multiple techniques from quantitative randomized controlled trials to in-depth qualitative explorations. Being able to draw from this continuum may allow answers to more complex and varied questions posed by commissioners and stakeholders at national and international level. In addition, these approaches can be combined, bringing further complexity to the process. Perhaps one of the most useful considerations of this type of research is presented by Robson (2011), who draws on Anastas and MacDonald's (1994) framework of fixed and flexible designs and argues that in applied settings fixed (or quantitative) designs require significant understanding in terms of the boundaries of the research, feasibility, etc., while flexible (or qualitative) designs allow for a more responsive research design that can respond to the challenges that may develop during the course of a study. For example, in research that cannot benefit from drawing on a large body of existing research, an initial qualitative study can provide important direction. A recent evaluation of the Barretstown therapeutic recreation programme for families affected by childhood cancer (www.barretstown.org) faced this specific challenge (see Box 6.2).

Box 6.2 Developing research in the absence of an existing body of research

Barretstown is a charity based in Kildare, Ireland, which aims to support children and families affected by serious childhood illness (see www.barretstown.org). The organization has been involved in several research projects designed to explore aspects of its programmes for children and families. One project involved supporting an evaluation of its family programme, but a question arose about the most appropriate outcomes to assess in this context. While there is a relatively large body of research on the impact of childhood cancer on the family, there is less on family-based intervention (Meyler, Guerin, Kiernan & Breatnach, 2010). In the absence of a clear empirical foundation, the researchers employed a small exploratory study (which used interviews with staff and parents) to identify the variables to be included in a larger quasi-experimental evaluation (Meyler, 2009). The findings of this initial study informed the way in which the research team refined the research question for the following evaluation. This allowed the researchers to be informed by specific experiences of the programme highlighted by the exploratory study in developing the eventual evaluation.

In addition to qualitative and quantitative research designs, researchers can also draw on the growing interest in mixed-methods research. Mixed-methods have been growing in popularity in recent times, and this approach has been described as a methodological revolution in health, social and behavioural sciences (Tashakkori & Teddlie, 1998). Many of the proponents argue that this approach is more than the simple combination of different studies to answer a research question (Tashakkori & Teddlie, 2003). Mixed-methods research involves seeing the strengths and limitations of more traditional approaches and using the strengths of one to offset the limitations of the other. It builds on a multi-method approach – by which several methods from within one (qualitative or quantitative) framework are combined – allowing a greater range of options in combining elements of the research design. Recognizing the complexity identified in real world and applied research, Robson (2011) argues for the use of mixed-method research designs. Indeed, some of these ideas have been observed in tenders by services and sites funded by The Atlantic Philanthropies and the Irish Office for the Minister of Children and Young People discussed in other chapters within this text. Reviewing international research tenders, similar patterns are evident. For example, a tender issued by Social Work Scotland included reference to use of existing data, surveys and focus groups to explore public attitudes towards social services (www.socialworkscotland.org/Home/Research-tender-opportunity), while a recent call issued for a study of health care in prison settings also specified the use of mixed-methods (https://kce.fgov.be/sites/default/files/page_documents/207693_en.pdf). The World Health Organization's (WHO) report on youth tobacco use recognizes these developments, and states that evaluations should use a combination of qualitative and quantitative methods (Mehl, Stimson, Riley & Ball, 2002).

Another factor that has impacted on the expectations among tenderers and host organizations is the growing interest in the discipline of implementation science and the increased awareness of this area (Glasgow et al., 2012). While the use of the randomized controlled trial (RCT) design has long been recognized as the so called 'gold standard' in evaluation and effectiveness research (Maclure, Carleton & Schneeweiss, 2007), its use in a large variety of settings and applications is not always appropriate or feasible. Readers may be more familiar with RCTs in medical and particularly pharmaceutical research; however, the design is increasingly being used in a wider variety of settings (see the Medical Research Council guidelines on the evaluation of complex health interventions, Campbell et al., 2000). Many of the calls for research influenced by the collaboration of The Atlantic Philanthropies and the Irish Department of Children and Youth Affairs discussed in this text have specified the combination of traditional RCTs with more qualitative process evaluations that seem to develop a deeper understanding of the patterns observed by the RCT elements. This sentiment is also expressed by the Chairperson of the National Institute for Health and Care Excellence (NICE) in the United Kingdom, who has stated that traditional hierarchies of evidence are overly simplistic and a diversity of approaches needs to be implemented (Rawlins, 2008). Rawlins points to the need for a more cognitive approach to evidence-based policymaking, and his comments mark a broader shift in thinking to recognize the importance of both experimental and non-experimental methods in comparative effectiveness research or 'CER'.

The CER approach is considered the new 'gold standard' in effectiveness research and has been endorsed and funded in the Health Reform Bill in the United States (Tunis, Benner & McClellen, 2010). At the centre of CER is meaningful engagement and feedback from local policy and service providers and the incorporation of a wide variety of relevant qualitative and quantitative research methodologies into policy and service provision decisions. Clearly this is one element of research design and implementation where effective engagement between the commissioners, hosts and researchers is key to the success of the research and its eventual relevance to practice. However, it is important that at the design stage the researchers have a clear sense of how these elements will be combined and that this approach has its own design conventions above and beyond those evident in qualitative and quantitative research.

Some of the challenges and possible solutions involved in designing research in real world community settings will be considered later in this chapter. However, before considering the elements of an applied design and indeed reflecting on these, a key principle that must be considered is rigour, or 'scientific rigour', as some researchers refer to it. The dominance of quantitative or experimental research rests on science's desire to study phenomena objectively (Shaughnessy, Zechmeister & Zechmeister, 2008). This allows the researcher to have more confidence in the extent to which the research is unbiased and does indeed tell us about the populations we are interested in (rather than just the sample of this group that has taken part in the research). However, applied research can sometimes be undermined by an assumption that all quantitative research is rigorous while qualitative research is inherently less so. This is not surprising when one recognizes that many researchers are trained in a particular approach.

However, challenges arise when researchers assume that the rigour of a study lies in the general approach taken rather than care taken in designing and implementing the study. It could be argued that rigour comes not from a particular design, but from recognizing the process as a piece of research and working to introduce as much rigour as is possible given the context of the research and the phenomena being studied. For example, an RCT of a community-based intervention can be undermined by problems with random allocation of participants, while a qualitative study can be enhanced through the use of a systematic sampling strategy that identifies the key groups central to the study and works to control the biases that may influence the selection process. Whatever the methodological approach favoured by the researchers, it is important to remember that the commissioners, hosts and other stakeholders may have needs for the resultant data and findings that influence this choice. For example, data in the form of figures on the use of or demand for services may allow a service to seek additional financial support from its funders, while qualitative stories of service users' experiences may allow the organization to present a clear and personal narrative of the work they do. Open discussion between commissioners and researchers can allow for these needs to be considered and addressed in the most effective way.

It is important to remember that applying the scientific method does not automatically make a study rigorous. A possible misnomer in real world research is the use of the adjective 'scientific'. Robson (2011) argues that perhaps it is better for research in these complex settings to aim to be systematic rather than scientific. Qualitative, quantitative and mixed-methods research should be conducted in a systematic fashion, with a clear rationale underpinning all key decisions in the research process. In addition, recognizing the potential for challenges in complex real world settings, it is also important that when researchers are responding to unanticipated challenges they are systematic in how they respond to them. The next section will consider some of these challenges and explore possible solutions.

Reflecting on the design process

Moving on to explore the process of designing a research study to be conducted in a real world setting in more detail, a useful overview of the process is provided by Hedrick, Bickman and Rog (1993). They see research in real world settings as consisting of four main stages: Definition (the development of the research question described above); Design and Planning; Implementation; and Reporting/Follow-up. They break Stage 2 – Design and Planning – down further into the following elements:

- Choose design and data collection approaches;
- Review the resources available;
- Assess the feasibility of the planned design;
- Identify the trade-offs necessary.

Many researchers will be familiar with these elements of the research process. However, funders/commissioners and users of research may not be aware of the choices to be made during the research process. Therefore, this model provides a useful framework within which to consider the questions and challenges that can arise in applied and community-based research. More importantly, it is possible to reflect on these challenges and explore possible solutions. Each of the four elements of Design and Planning should be considered from a perspective of the implications for research design in real world settings.

In terms of *choosing the design and data collection approaches* to be used, we have already highlighted that researchers working in applied and community settings should be open to drawing from a range of approaches to design. In addition, the research question must be the central influence in the process of design. However, there are several issues that must be considered at this point. To begin, the researchers must consider if there is a particular design specified in the tender or funding document, or more likely if there are particular principles specified (e.g. representativeness). As noted earlier, many of the projects funded under the Irish Prevention and Early Intervention Programme (PEIP) which is considered in several other chapters in this text specified the need for RCT-based evaluation and process evaluation elements. Another example was evident in a tender published by the National Disability Authority in Ireland that called for the selection of a nationally representative sample of people with disabilities. This pattern is also evident internationally. For example, a tender issued by the UK charity Nesta (www.nesta.org.uk) to evaluate its 'People Powered Results Programme' requested both a quantitative assessment of outcomes and a qualitative process evaluation, while guidelines issued by the Government of Western Australia outline the use of both approaches in public health research (Program Evaluation Unit, 2015).

Whatever the preferences held by the funder or commissioner, clearly publicized requirements and expectations are in all parties' best interests. However, challenges can arise when these requirements or principles are not made explicit. Depending on the individuals or groups involved in drafting a tender or deciding the focus of a call for funding, it is possible that there are different levels of experience and familiarity informing this process, an issue considered in Chapter 3 in greater detail. It is important for the researchers to gather as much information as possible on these expectations and preferences related to the possible design of the research, either in the form of the publically available documentation or other negotiations with the funder or key organization. Following on from this, the research team must reflect on their own orientation and, more practically, the expertise they have access to. Challenges can arise when a research team fails to appreciate the intricacies of the project at hand. For example, a team with a predominantly quantitative or experimental orientation may not appreciate the complexity of an action research design. However, one of the simplest solutions to this challenge is collaboration, with the research team inviting researchers with the required expertise to work on the project.

Moving on to the specific methods of data collection, the options will again be defined by both the question and the design chosen. For example, if the question relates to the effectiveness of an intervention and a randomized controlled trial has been selected, then the researchers may consider the use of questionnaires or formal observation. Both methods of data collection require that the concepts being studied have been operationalized (e.g. reading ability is operationalized as scores on a standardized test of reading aptitude, or community safety is operationalized as self-reported responses to a series of questions on perceived personal safety). It is also possible that the research question will have more than one component (as discussed in the opening section above), and these different components may each require different methods of data collection. It is important at this stage that the researchers identify a range of options, as the following phases of the research process (outlined in the Hedrick et al. model above) will influence the choices made.

Having chosen a possible research design and selected options for data collection, it is important that the researchers then *review the resources available*. Research is a resource intensive process, whether in the form of the funding available for the project, the time allocated by different members of the research team and/or the organizations supporting the project. In-kind resources may not be factored into the budget, but the willingness of all parties to contribute time and knowledge can significantly influence the outcomes of the research and its eventual value to the organization, representing important added value for all parties involved. Hedrick et al. (1993) also stress the need to consider the information resources required by the project. For example, a research team may plan to draw on existing data held by the organization, but a lack of understanding of the process and time involved in accessing the data in a useful manner and format may involve a commitment of time and resources that limit the return from including it.

In recent years, the process of budgeting for a research project has become more challenging. The appointment of research staff is made more complex by the impact of employment legislation and legal entitlements to paid holidays, pension contributions and redundancy contributions. Other funding issues researchers must be aware of include whether a piece of research is liable for value added tax (VAT), which is applied to goods and services in many countries, and whether the host institution requires a contribution towards indirect overheads in research funding. These issues require research teams to be familiar with these issues and aware of them when developing budgets, or more feasibly having access to supports within their home organization to advise on these requirements. It is also important that funders/commissioners are aware that these may be legitimate expenses that researchers, particularly those in academic settings, may be required to include in the budget for the project. Increasingly, university research offices/departments provide resources to staff to assist in developing budgets. In Ireland, the Irish Universities Association have issued guidelines on salary scales for researcher posts, with information included on mandatory and optional contributions such as pension and redundancy (www.iua.ie/research-innovation/researcher-salary-scales/). In addition, major granting bodies such as the US National Institutes of Health provide comprehensive advice for researchers that can also be helpful for commissioners of research (https://grants.nih.gov/grants/how-to-apply-application-guide/format-and-write/develop-your-budget.htm).

According to the model guiding this chapter, the next element of the research design process involves *assessing the feasibility of the planned design*. There are many elements of a design that must be considered in terms of feasibility. An obvious one relates to the resources allocated for the project, but this involves a consideration of the resources that others must bring to the project. For example, as mentioned above, the sourcing of secondary data and other information may require a significant input by the organization in which the research is being conducted. It is important that the research team can give the organization a clear idea of the work involved. However, if the research project is the focus of a competitive tender, there may be limited time to establish this information in advance of submitting a tender. Where the project is being developed as a collaborative piece of work between a research team and a community setting, it will be easier for the research team to establish the feasibility of key elements of the design.

Another important aspect of feasibility is knowing the setting or the community in which the research will take place. Again, this can be less problematic when developing a collaborative project, or when the research team has experience of working in the setting previously. A significant challenge to feasibility and design is the issue of expected response rates. Designing a quantitative study that relies on an adequate sample size to ensure the power of the statistical analyses is often based on assumptions about response rates. However, researchers who have experience of working in less controlled settings, such as communities, may not have an accurate insight into the response rates that may be expected. In terms of responding to this issue, practical solutions include reviewing previous research conducted with the specific group or similar groups to identify a feasible response rate, calculating required response rates allowing for conservative rates of participant loss or attrition, and working with the organizations in the setting, such as schools and community groups, to maximize the participation rates. When reviewing feasibility, the most useful tool available to the research team is a comprehensive pilot study. A preliminary trial of the research procedure and instruments will highlight some of the potential challenges and allow the researchers to identify solutions.

Related to feasibility is the task of *identifying the trade-offs necessary* to ensure the successful completion of the research. It is important that a research team know the elements of the research that can vary and those that are central to the study and therefore cannot change. Hedrick et al. (1993) discuss the range of factors that could influence these trade-offs, including the aforementioned resource limitations. One key issue they discuss in terms of identifying trade-offs relates to the external generalizability of the study. As mentioned earlier, one of the challenges of research design in real world and community settings is the need to balance rigour and feasibility. For example, conducting an evaluation of an after-school programme in a community setting may mean that the findings are more relevant to the population of interest. However, it does raise challenges to the internal validity or experimental control of the evaluation. Another possible trade-off may occur in multi-site studies. A clear benefit of using multi-site studies is the potential for larger sample sizes and more powerful analyses. However, the inclusion of multiple service providers and multiple contexts creates more room for confounding variables and nuisance factors.

Conclusion

When reviewing the elements of the development of a research design in a complex real-world setting, several key lessons have emerged. The first relates to knowing the setting and the key stakeholders in the research to be completed. This knowledge will allow the researchers to make informed design decisions and to carry out an effective evaluation of the resources and trade-offs involved in the planning process. It is also important to remember that the stakeholders will play multiple roles in the research process. Stakeholders may be funders, gatekeepers, facilitators, participants and the consumers of the final product. It is also important to remember that real world and community research generally involves a diverse range of stakeholders with varying levels of familiarity and trust of research and researchers. Again, understanding the context and the parties involved is central to the researchers' successful engagement during the design process. While the success of the funding application or tender may be out of the researchers' hands, it is important to remember that it is the beginning of a process. Identifying and solving problems successfully at this phase will lead to a stronger plan for the implementation stage of research. Perhaps the key lesson when designing research in a real world community setting is to realize that a study that is well designed, well communicated and meets the needs of the full range of stakeholders is but the first step in the process, and that a well-designed study should enable, suggest and encourage further valuable research of relevance to the community and the researcher.

References

Anastas, J.W. & MacDonald, M.L. (1994) *Research design for social work and the human services.* New York, NY: Lexington Books.

Campbell, M., Fitzpatrick, R., Haines, A., Kinmonth, A.L., Sandercock, P., Spiegelhalter, D. & Tyrer, P. (2000) 'Framework for design and evaluation of complex interventions to improve health', *British Medical Journal*, 321, pp. 694–696.

Comiskey, C.M., Kelly, P., Leckey, Y., McCulloch, L., O'Duill, B., Stapleton, R.D. & White, E. (2009) *The ROSIE study – Drug treatment outcomes in Ireland.* Dublin: The Stationery Office, Government Publications.

Glasgow, R.E., Vinson, C., Chambers, D., Khoury, M.J., Kaplan, R.M. & Hunter, C. (2012) 'National Institutes of Health approaches to dissemination and implementation science: Current and future directions', *American Journal of Public Health*, 102(7), pp. 1274–1281.

Hedrick, T.E., Bickman, L. & Rog, D.J. (1993) *Applied research design: A practical guide.* Thousand Oaks, CA: SAGE.

Hubbard, R. L., Craddock, S.G. & Anderson, J. (2003) 'Overview of five-year follow-up outcomes in the Drug Abuse Treatment Outcome Studies (DATOS)', *Journal of Substance Abuse Treatment*, 25(3), pp. 125–134.

Jones, A., Donmall, M., Millar, T., Moody, A., Weston, S., Anderson, T., Gittins, M., Abeywardana, V. & D'Souza, J. (2009) *The drug treatment outcomes research study: Final outcomes report.* London: Home Office.

Maclure, M., Carleton, B. & Schneeweiss, S. (2007) 'Designed delays versus rigorous pragmatic trials: lower carat gold standards can produce relevant, drug evaluations', *Medical Care*, 45(10), pp. S44–S49.

Mehl, G., Stimson, V.G., Riley, L. & Ball, A. (2002) *Youth tobacco – Rapid assessment and response guide.* Version 1.0. Geneva: World Health Organization.

Meyler, E. (2009) *Mitigating the impact of childhood cancer on Irish families: The role of therapeutic recreation.* PhD Thesis submitted to University College Dublin.

Meyler, E., Guerin, S.Kiernan, G. & Breatnach, L. (2010) 'A review of family based psychosocial interventions for families affected by childhood cancer', *Journal of Paediatric Psychology*, 35(10), pp. 1116–1132.

Program Evaluation Unit (2015) *Evaluation guide.* Perth: Department of Treasury, Government of Western Australia.

Rawlins, M. (2008) 'De testimonio: On the evidence for decisions about the use of therapeutic interventions', *Lancet*, 372, pp. 2152–2161.

Robson, C. (2011) *Real world research.* Malden, MA: Blackwell.

Shaughnessy, J., Zechmeister, E. & Zechmeister, J. (2008) *Research methods in psychology.* 8th edn. New York, NY: McGraw Hill.

Tashakkori, A. & Teddlie, C. (2003) *Handbook of mixed methods in social and behavioural research.* Thousand Oaks, CA: SAGE.

Tashakkori, A. & Teddlie, C. (1998) *Mixed methodology: Combining qualitative and quantitative approaches.* Thousand Oaks, CA: SAGE.

Teesson, M. *et al.* (2006) 'One year outcomes for heroin dependence: Findings from the Australian Treatment Outcome Study (ATOS)', *Drug and Alcohol Dependence*, 83(2), pp. 174–180.

Tunis, S.R., Benner, J. & McClellan, M. (2010) 'Comparative effectiveness research: Policy context, methods development and research infrastructure', *Statistics in Medicine*, 29(19), pp. 1963–1976.

7 What lies beneath? Preparing for and conducting effective fieldwork in community settings

Tara Murphy, Jennie Milnes and Siobhán Keegan

Introduction

Community-based research often draws on multiple methods and approaches in order to gather high quality quantitative and qualitative data from a variety of sources. While the nature and purpose of these studies vary, almost all require a team of competent and reliable fieldworkers to gather data across differing contexts and populations. Researchers tend to overlook (or underestimate) the benefits and potential learning of reporting the organization and implementation of the fieldwork phase of studies. Much of the social sciences literature emphasizes the methodological and analytic approaches used by researchers, with less attention being paid to the pragmatic and process issues associated with research, for example, the competencies of fieldworkers who gather the data, the delivery of fieldwork training by those leading the research, the type of support fieldworkers are offered throughout the data collection process or the potential way fieldworkers' perceptions and experiences may influence participants' responses. Indeed, much of the fieldwork process has to be inferred by the readers. Studies that describe the selection, recruitment and training of fieldworkers tend to employ various definitions of fieldwork from 'fieldworker in research' to 'fieldworker in practice', and are more likely to be ethnographic or anthropologic in nature.

This chapter argues that understanding what lies beneath data is as important as knowing the outcomes of research. Previous research highlights the correlation between the quality of the data analysis and how well the data are collected (Gregory & Radovinsky, 2012; Kitto, Chester & Grbich, 2008). Poorly gathered data may be misleading or misinterpreted and result in the development of inappropriate policies and practices. Similarly, they may have a negative impact in terms of research ethics (as discussed in Chapter 4). The purpose of this chapter is to elucidate some of the key issues pertaining to planning for and conducting fieldwork, particularly in relation to the recruitment and training of fieldworkers and the potential for fieldwork behaviour to influence participants' responses, and it identifies some of the practicalities of conducting fieldwork with vulnerable groups, including children. 'Fieldworkers', 'data collectors', 'surveyors', 'research workers' and 'interviewers' are used interchangeably by various studies depending on the nature of the research. This chapter will use the term 'fieldworker' to refer to all those responsible for gathering data in a research setting.

Real world research poses additional and oftentimes complex challenges for researchers, as evidenced throughout this book. These include entry into a community, managing expectations and relationships between key stakeholders, dealing with competing agendas and engaging with different populations. As a result, fieldworkers undertaking community-based fieldwork may be required to adhere to more rigorous data collection protocols and procedures compared with their laboratory based counterparts (Jensen, Hoagwood & Trickett, 1999). This chapter draws on both the international literature as well as the experience of the authors in order to provide readers with a very practical insight into the recruitment, selection, training and supporting of fieldworkers.

Recruitment, selection and training of fieldworkers

Recruitment and selection

Fieldworkers may be recruited in several ways, for example, by gaining prior permission from another researcher to access his/her pool of fieldworkers, advertising via postgraduate notice boards and online discussion forums, or through more formal routes such as academic schools/departments. For more community-based participatory research, fieldworkers may be accessed at community meetings, through organizations that work closely with members of the community, by advertising in local newspapers or through social networking sites. Research undertaken by Green and Baxen (2002) found that the most common practices for hiring fieldworkers were personal contact, networking, accessing pools of fieldworkers and advertising.

Researchers may have different criteria for selecting fieldworkers, depending largely on the nature and purpose of the research project. Qualitative research studies (with individual interviews and focus groups, for example) require fieldworkers with highly developed listening, interpersonal, and communication skills (Marshall & Rossman, 1995, cited in Green & Baxen, 2002). Being able to interpret verbal and non-verbal responses, probing participants where appropriate and knowing how to ask sensitive questions (e.g. on mental health, household income and family issues) are important skills that fieldworkers should own. Possessing specific academic qualifications or technical knowledge may be important in circumstances where the research involves psychometric and biomedical testing.

It may be considered important that fieldworkers are familiar with the sociocultural and environmental context of the target population, which may in turn enhance data integrity (Green & Baxen, 2002; Smith, 2008; True, Alexander & Richman, 2011). There are several advantages to recruiting fieldworkers who are from similar backgrounds to the research participants. For example, participants may be more willing to disclose information to someone they perceive as being from a similar background. There may also be greater engagement in the research from participants. Fieldworkers themselves may feel more comfortable in a particular setting. However, it is equally important to consider the potentially undesirable effects that may occur in the recruitment of fieldworkers from within the target population, including the risk of attrition due to fieldworkers feeling overburdened, the increased potential for missing or inaccurate data, lack of experience among fieldworkers of this type of work and, in some cases, difficulty maintaining confidentiality – all of which have the potential to undermine the integrity of the data as well as threaten research ethics (True, Alexander & Richman, 2011). A study carried out by Alexander and Richman (2008) examined fieldwork undertaken by former drug users with existing drug users. They found that this group of fieldworkers faced a high risk of relapse during the data collection process as a consequence of being re-exposed to drugs, which had ethical and moral implications for lead researchers. Fieldworkers may also unintentionally bias participants' responses or adapt the way in which they pose particular questions depending on who the participants are (Smith, 2008). In some cases, participants may refuse to participate in the research for the simple reason that they know or are familiar with the fieldworker.

According to Babbie (1990), fieldworkers undertaking qualitative research may unduly influence the quality and outcome of the data. An evaluation report by Bjørkhaug, Perdersen and Bøås (2007) on the living conditions of individuals with disabilities in Zambia hypothesized that in terms of the accuracy of the study's findings, "the quality of the response suffers, because the interaction between [fieldworkers] and respondent may lead to either over- or under-communication of the degree of disability, depending on how sympathy and views on relative disability develop between the interviewer and respondent" (p. 11). Fowler (2002) estimates that up to half of participants' responses in most surveys may be affected or influenced by fieldworkers, which is worrying. This highlights the importance of training and ongoing supervision of fieldworkers to minimize this potential threat. A similar phenomenon, social desirability, is considered in more detail later in this chapter. It too has the potential to affect participant responses and undermine data integrity. Other practical issues to consider during the selection process are fieldworkers' availability during the data collection period, convenience in terms of their distance from the fieldwork setting and access to private transport, which may be an essential pre-requisite for studies conducted in several distant locations.

In most circumstances fieldworkers will be incentivized to gather data. Ideally these incentives will be commensurate with the task at hand, though this is not always possible when there are limited resources available to the researcher. True, Alexander and Richman (2011) found that fieldworkers who perceived an incentive or award to be unfair or insufficient were more likely to engage in research misbehaviour in the form of, for example, fabricating completed surveys or participants' responses to specific questions. Where resources are available, fieldworkers may benefit in terms of monetary, professional or altruistic recompense. For example, the lead author paid fieldworkers €20 per hour to participate in fieldwork training and €10 per completed survey, with the requirement that a minimum of 10 completed surveys were gathered prior to payment for training. This was a precautionary measure employed by the researcher in order to reduce the likelihood of attrition during and after the training sessions. Regardless of the type of incentive available, it is imperative that those interested in training as fieldworkers have a clear understanding of the purpose and nature of the research, have clear expectations and are aware of the commitment necessary for completing specific tasks. This may minimize the potential for attrition among fieldworkers as the research progresses. Once the recruitment and selection process is complete, fieldworkers participate in appropriate training to develop their skills and increase their competence in undertaking ethically sound and reliable data collection.

Training fieldworkers

The delivery of high quality fieldwork training including booster training is critical to ensuring the collection of reliable data (Smith, 2008). Achieving and maintaining quality assurance in terms of surveys or interviews is an important though difficult task (Grosh & Glewwe, 2000). Though there are ways to monitor data integrity – for example, examining quality indicators such as the prevalence of non-responses or estimates of standard errors – training fieldworkers is likely to enhance the quality of the data. Therefore, training offered to fieldworkers should be sufficient so as to allow fieldworkers gain sufficient understanding of the purpose and nature of the research, long enough to allow for repeated practice and the development of key skills and offer several opportunities for some experiential learning (Babbie, 1990; Fowler, 2002; Grosh & Glewwe, 2000).

Üstun et al. (2003) emphasize the importance of training fieldworkers in order to ensure quality data collection. They posit that training increases the likelihood that fieldworkers will become more engaged in the research process, implement questions or instruments reliably and gain further insight into the research participants. The current authors propose several additional reasons for training fieldworkers, including ensuring the fieldwork is conducted in an ethical manner, increasing the capacity of fieldworkers to overcome challenges in the field by problem-solving and developing a mutually trusting relationship with fieldworkers.

In terms of models of fieldwork training, Green and Baxen (2002) proposed three models of training which are briefly described now. The 'Engagement' model is similar to the action or participatory research model, where the researcher engages with the fieldworker within the fieldworker's context (e.g. members of the community becoming fieldworkers and conducting fieldwork within their community). This model involves an intensive process of self-reflection in which both the researcher and the fieldworker reflect on the work they are undertaking as part of the research process. There is also acknowledgement of the inherent strengths fieldworkers possess in terms of knowledge of the field and specific skills (Green & Baxen, 2002).

A second model of fieldwork training is the 'Mentorship' model, whereby senior researchers mentor fieldworkers by working alongside them, demonstrating skills and providing valuable opportunities for reciprocal and experiential learning.

A third model of training is the 'Partnership' model, where the researcher and fieldworker work in partnership in order to conduct effective fieldwork. Both partners share equal responsibilities in terms of overseeing the implementation of the fieldwork. It is a balanced relationship with a shared set of roles, tasks and decision-making responsibilities.

In designing and delivering a fieldwork training programme, lead researchers may consider an interactive, experiential format rather than a didactic one, to allow fieldworkers the opportunity to develop a deeper understanding of the experience of being a research participant. This role playing or 'in their shoes' approach may incorporate the use of vignettes where fieldworkers engage in a blinded role play, with one fieldworker being provided with a vignette that may reflect the background of a research participant (demographics, family history, substance use, etc.) and the other fieldworker administering the questionnaire without any knowledge of the vignette. In pairs, potential fieldworkers may take it in turns to administer the questionnaires, then feed back to their partner on the experience of this before reversing roles, with the interviewer becoming the participant. Feedback may take place again in pairs and then to the wider group, with fieldworkers summarizing their experience of being the participant and responding to the questionnaires. Modifications may be made to the research protocol where any issues arise, though careful consideration should be given to standardized questionnaires and inter-rater consistency in the research protocol. Following modifications, a similar review process may be undertaken prior to fieldwork commencing. Table 7.1 provides sample case studies which were used by fieldworkers in a community research needs analysis study to explore a variety of data collection scenarios (Murphy & Guerin, 2012). Finally, it is also recommended that more fieldworkers are trained than necessary to compensate for potential attrition over the course of the research study.

Doing fieldwork: Practical concerns

Fieldwork with any group has certain associated practicalities, many of which do not receive much research attention. This section outlines some of the main practicalities and considerations associated with conducting fieldwork, which should be covered in training and included in fieldwork protocols.

Table 7.1 Sample case studies with some solutions

Scenario	*Solutions*
1) The participant answers the door and you are suddenly tongue-tied!	✓ Apologize. ✓ Return to the interview script and start again! ✓ Preparation is important – remember practice makes perfect (or nearly)!
2) You are unfamiliar with the area you have chosen but are looking forward to getting to know the area and meeting new people. You randomly select the first house and knock on the door. There is no response. The next four randomly selected houses are also empty. You arrive at the sixth randomly selected house and a mother answers the door holding a crying baby.	✓ Briefly explain the purpose of the call. ✓ Leave the information sheet. ✓ Reschedule to do the survey at a more convenient time.
3) The participant is very interested in the survey and is happy to answer all questions. You enjoy the openness of the conversation until the participant starts to wander off on tangents for 5–10 minutes each. You find it difficult to 'control' the conversation and are beginning to grow weary.	✓ Be patient! ✓ Listen to the participant and try to direct him/her back to the question by drawing out the key messages from what they have stated. ✓ Inform the participant that s/he will have an opportunity to elaborate later in the survey. ✓ Introduce a little bit of light-heartedness (e.g. 'Oh my, would you look at the time. We should get back to the survey or else I'll be here for tea time!').
4) The participant offers to make you a cup of tea and you're sitting there at the kitchen table enjoying the interview process when suddenly you see the participant give his/her child a hard slap.	✓ Remember – you have a duty of care to report any issues relating to child protection and you will have stated this from the outset. ✓ Assess the situation (e.g. how hard was the slap? Where did the child receive the slap? What were the circumstances?). ✓ Stay calm. ✓ Do not judge the participant. ✓ Continue with the survey if appropriate. ✓ Complete the incident log sheet once you leave the house. ✓ Discuss the situation with CDI immediately.

Scenario	*Solutions*
5) You are right in the middle of asking the first of several 'sensitive' questions when the participant says "Sorry, this survey is becoming too personal. Why are you asking me these types of questions? What are you going to do with the information?" The participant becomes frustrated and asks if you are checking up on them on behalf of someone else.	✓ Remind the participant that you are not from the social services, social welfare or local authority. ✓ Reassure the participant by reminding them about anonymity and confidentiality (e.g. who will see the information; how it will be stored; etc.). ✓ Remind the participant about the overall purpose of the survey and how the information will be used. ✓ Invite him/her to complete the questions/that section by hand. ✓ Be respectful of their final decision.
6) The person refuses to take part in the study and tells you in no uncertain terms to "go away"! You're upset and want to throw it all in.	✓ Remain professional. ✓ Thank the individual (yes, really!). ✓ De-brief with your fieldwork partner and/or CDI. ✓ Remember – it's not about you! The individual may be having a bad day and you caught him/her at the wrong time!

Fieldwork protocols

The clue to one of the most important and basic practicalities of fieldwork is in the name: It is work that happens in the field, that is, somewhere that is possibly new to the fieldworker and will most likely require travel to get there. Inexperienced fieldworkers can fail by focusing on the intricacies of fieldwork and forgetting the basic practicalities. (Where am I going, how do I get there, are they expecting me and what will they expect *of* me?) The development of written fieldwork protocols to cover the myriad eventualities that may occur in the field is advisable. A protocol is defined as "the accepted or established code of procedure or behaviour in any group, organization, or situation". The development of fieldwork protocols is essential for any research team to ensure the uniform and reliable collection of data, particularly when multiple sites and fieldworkers are involved. They should be used as a training tool during fieldworker training and a written copy should be provided to fieldworkers before they leave to begin fieldwork. If protocols are overlooked, data collection in the field may be compromised. The following are some of the key areas for consideration when conducting fieldwork in community settings:

- fieldworker self-reflexivity and awareness;
- social desirability;
- organizational protocols (location information, contact details, schedule, materials);
- fieldworker safety and well-being;
- ethics (meaningful assent and participant understanding of research), which is discussed in Chapter 4.

Fieldworker self-reflexivity

Fieldworkers need to constantly examine and re-examine the power relationship between themselves and their participants. This requires the ability to reflect honestly on themselves and the events in which they are involved. It is important that a fieldworker gives some prior consideration to how a participant is likely to view them and that they take steps to avoid reinforcing any negative suspicions they are likely to have (Sluka, 1990). Physical appearance can be an important consideration when conducting fieldwork. It is important that fieldworkers do not differentiate themselves unduly from the research population through ostentatious clothing, jewellery, equipment or belongings (Goldstein, 2014). Physical cues denoting difference between the fieldworkers and participants can engender feelings of resentment, anxiety or distraction and may lead to lack of engagement with the research process and increased risk of theft or attack (Goldstein, 2014). Barker and Weller (2003) discuss the importance of considering 'geography' when conducting research with children, for example. In schools, children know that they are expected to do what an adult asks of them (Morrow & Richards, 1996). They are also expected to have the right answer, so watchful fieldworkers should notice if children are trying to provide the right answer or a quick answer rather than their real answer. It can be useful to remind and reassure children that there are no right or wrong answers.

Research studies (Corsaro, 2005; Waller & Bitou, 2011) have noted how physical factors (such as body size or facial hair) and social factors (power roles among adults and children) often mean that children have trouble differentiating a researcher from the other adults in their lives, that is, from seeing them as an 'atypical adult', which can have implications for the expectations children have about the research. In order to engage young children, therefore, it may be advisable for researchers to follow Warming's (2005) advice that a researcher move in and out of a 'child-like position' to differentiate her role from the normal adult. Unless a child is in danger, fieldworkers working with children should let infringements of the rules pass without note to demonstrate to the child that they do not have the same expectations of them as their parents and teachers. Ebrahim and Muthukrishna (2005) similarly advocate the adoption of intersecting roles within the researcher identity when researching with the under fours and the benefits of adopting a flexible identity (maternal, friendly, fun, positive) for the research process.

Indeed, flexibility of role seems to be key for adult populations also. Fieldworkers should be provided with the tools to engage flexibly with the research population at no cost to themselves. For example, a phone should be provided to help them to engage with the population, to arrange and re-schedule data collection and to link them back to their supervisory team. Watchful fieldworkers will notice when a participant is disengaged and implement strategies to ameliorate that, such as taking a break, increasing the energy in their body language or voice or perhaps ceasing the research altogether.

Awareness also improves the quality of the data collected through the addition of a more finely tuned interpretive layer to the data. It involves developing an explicit awareness of what might otherwise be taken for granted (Bernard, 2006; Goldstein, 2014). It can be useful to suggest that fieldworkers keep a data collection diary to make note of any relevant happenings in the field that might have an impact on the results. In a recent study, one of the current authors noted that a child had under-performed for their age on a spatial relations task involving the building of mirrored block structures, by placing them very far to one side instead of directly in front of them. The field notes indicated that the child wore an eyepatch, which meant that the child's ability to centre objects was negatively affected by the eyepatch. Therefore, the child's score on that test was not used, as it did not reflect an accurate portrayal of their spatial relations ability.

The issue of social desirability

Social desirability (SD) refers to the idea that there is a tendency for people to over-report behaviours and attitudes that comply with social norms (Kreuter, Presser & Tourangeau, 2008), while under-reporting or minimizing behaviours which do not comply with social norms. Socially desirable responding (SDR) confounds research results by creating false relationships or obscuring relationships between variables, and research studies have found evidence to show that SDR is prevalent in research participants' responses, regardless of age (van de Mortel, 2009). The ways in which fieldworkers elicit information from research participants can impact on the degree to which SDR is present, and plays an important role in ensuring the integrity of data. Inaccurate data may be misleading, and while researchers cannot exclusively or ultimately control participant responses, their awareness of and sensitivity to the questions that they are asking, their level of skills and training in conducting interviews and their ability to administer questionnaires effectively – all in a setting that is conducive to safe disclosure – play an important role in contributing to data integrity. Just as social workers, nurses, psychologists and other health professionals are trained to develop their skills and awareness of these, it can be argued that those conducting research in the community can benefit from training which incorporates a basic knowledge and awareness of social desirability.

Some research questions are considered more sensitive than others, and are more likely to trigger SDR. According to Tourangeau and Yan (2007), if respondents perceive research questions as intrusive, or if questions raise fears about potential repercussions of disclosing the information, SDR is more likely. The kinds of questions that may be considered sensitive are wide and varied, and depend often on the population being researched, the setting in which the research takes place, and the relationship of the research team to, for example, statutory services. Some examples of research topics commonly considered sensitive include drug and alcohol use, sexual health and activity, parenting (including children's physical and mental health), diet and exercise, personal hygiene habits, relationships with or custody of children, forensic history and financial background/income.

Adolescents have been found to provide SD responses to sensitive research topics. In a randomized controlled trial (RCT) of more than 1,200 male and female students aged between 15 and 21 years, van Griensven et al. (2006) tested the impact of data collection using palm-top assisted self-interviewing, audio computer-assisted self-interviewing, self-administered questionnaires and face-to-face interviews in combination with drug use urine testing. The results showed that self-administered questionnaires and computerized and audio-assisted questionnaire responses were superior to interviewer-administered questionnaires in collecting sensitive behavioural data, including sexual intercourse experience, oral sex, buying and selling sex, alcohol use, dietary behaviours, symptoms of depression and suicidal ideation. Overall, the more intimate or recent the sensitive behaviour, the more likely the respondent is to deny or minimise this in a face-to-face interview.

Similarly, adult participants have been shown to under-report socially undesirable behaviours, such as drinking alcohol (Davis, Thake & Vilhena, 2010) and illicit drug use (Tourangeau & Yan, 2007), and to over-report socially desirable behaviours, such as physical activity and physical activity durations (Adams et al., 2005) as well as socially desirable eating behaviours, such as eating fruit and vegetables (Hebert et al., 2008). Research with younger children too has found that food energy intake reporting was affected by the SD bias (Guinn et al., 2008; Guinn et al., 2010), with research showing that as social desirability increases, the reporting of food intake decreases.

It is crucial that researchers are aware of, and account for, the possibility of SDR throughout the research process. Community-based data collection with a deficit focus (i.e. gathering information on individual, family or community problems or deficits) which uses self-report measures is particularly methodologically vulnerable to elicit SD responding from participants (Crutzen & Goritz, 2010) and there is an opportunity here to consider ways in which community-based research can be designed to minimize the potential for SD responding.

Minimizing social desirability response (SDR)

Although SDR is often cited as the most common bias to affect community-based research, little information has been published about *how* researchers can address the issue of SDR during the various stages of a research project. One strategy is to measure social desirability by incorporating an SD scale into the research questionnaire (van de Mortel, 2009). The most widely used instrument to measure SD responding is the thirty-three item Marlowe Crowne Social Desirability Scale (Crown & Marlowe, 1960), in which the participant answers 'true' or 'false' to a set of socially desirable but improbable statements. Researchers can then use the scores from the SD scale to measure the degree to which participants are concerned with social approval.

Another strategy is to consider fieldworker (interviewer) behavior, and data collection methods (van Griensven et al., 2006). While self-administered questionnaires tend to yield increased rates of reporting information socially undesirable information (Kreuter et al., 2008), literacy issues, comprehension difficulties, computer skills (in the case of computerized assessment) and return rates suggest that self-administration of questionnaires by research participants is less favourable than interviewer-administered questionnaires. Where researchers decide on the use of fieldworker-administered interview style questionnaires, some training and experience in the use of indirect questioning is advised. Fisher (1993) examined the effects of asking indirect (structured, projective) questions, compared with direct (structured, personal) questions, and found that indirect questioning reduced SDR. Researchers involved in designing and developing studies must strike a delicate balance between the possible use of standardized questionnaires, providing fieldworkers with core training in interview/facilitation skills, which may yield richer, more accurate responses, while ensuring that interview and questionnaire protocols do not become too lengthy and cumbersome for participants.

The authors recommend that lead researchers design and deliver fieldworker training programmes which encourage and generate discussion among fieldworkers in considering the potential for SDR under the following key areas, encouraging fieldworkers to reflect on and consider:

- the research participants (for example general population or a target group such as drug users, migrants, sex workers or a cohort from a disadvantaged area), including factors such as:
    - cultural norms (values, family structure, gender roles, childrearing, diet);
    - gender norms (male female roles and expectations);
    - health norms (teeth cleaning, diet);
    - behaviour norms (monogamy in marriage);
- nature of questions that are being asked (*what* is being asked, *why*, and *by whom*);
- method of data collection being used (interviewer administered questionnaires *vs* independently completed online questionnaires, etc.);
- the setting in which the fieldwork will take place (participants' homes, on the street, in a statutory setting such as a school or a health service).

Finally, researchers may wish to consider the use of collateral (where appropriate) in the data collection process, for example, self-report plus urinalysis, self-report plus collateral from others, direct observation of behaviours, or the use of blood tests or physical activity monitors, where appropriate.

Fieldworker safety and well-being

Fieldworkers who work in the field can be exposed to a wide range or risks (Bahn & Weatherill, 2013). These risks include being exposed to emotionally challenging or upsetting information (Corbin & Morse, 2003; Mitchell & Irvine, 2008); risks to personal safety brought about by collecting data in a person's home (Lee, 1995); physical risk of contracting diseases when working with sick populations (Peterson, 2000); and safety risks when working with hard-to-reach groups such as drug dealers or prostitutes or in high-crime areas (Belousov et al., 2007; Bloor et al., 2010; Sampson & Thomas, 2003). Research suggests that fieldworker safety and wellbeing during research may be overlooked by those who supervise and hold grants for research projects (Bloor, Fincham & Sampson, 2010; Bahn, 2012; Tolbert, 2005). It is likely that if the risk is ancillary to the research question, it is easier for supervisors and institutions to overlook it, for example, if the research focuses on the early childhood care and education experiences of young children without due recognition of the fact that many of the children live in a high-crime location and have one or more parents involved in drug use. To overlook such risks has the effect of magnifying the danger for fieldworkers, according to Hopkins (2005).

Hubbard, Backett-Milburn and Kemmer (2001) posit that research supervisors are unlikely to have collected data themselves in many years and thus tend to forget or neglect the risks that may be encountered in the field. Bloor, Fincham and Sampson (2010) theorize that the lack of focus on risk to field-workers is a question of institutional culture. The institutional tendency to focus on ethical concerns for participants may have resulted in fieldworker safety and well-being staying out of focus at an institutional policy level. Bloor et al. (2010) report that in the UK tight research budgets are being blamed for the fact that academic institutions such as universities do not always implement safe working practices for fieldworkers. The implication is that the cost of practices such as paired working or systematic calls before and after is prohibitive for grant seekers who are under pressure from funders to submit competitive funding bids. If this is the case, it may be incumbent on grant holders to highlight the need for expenditure on fieldworker safety in research budget proposals and, in turn, for funders to provide the means to ensure that such safety precautions can become a reality. Bahn (2012) suggests that protecting fieldworkers from risk would benefit institutions financially in the long term. She contends that there is a financial relationship between managing risk and profitability, which applies to universities as much as to other institutions, and that the benefit accrued to institutions by minimizing risks should have financial (fewer claims, less staff illness) as well as altruistic benefits.

Strategies to support fieldworker safety

Paterson, Gregory and Thorne (1999) recommended general guidelines around developing a fieldworker safety protocol to prevent and avoid dangerous incidents in the course of research. Many institutions now require a risk assessment and risk management strategy to be completed prior to fieldwork commencement (Corbin & Morse, 2003). However, there is some evidence, both from literature and anecdotally, that these often standardized assessments fall short of asking the relevant questions needed to ensure the safety and well-being of researchers in areas such as the social sciences (Bahn, 2012; Dickson-Swift, James & Kippen, 2007).

One of the most important factors for ensuring fieldworker safety and well-being is advance planning, according to Paterson and colleagues. While it is well documented that piloting of research instruments can be useful for instrument refinement, Sampson (2004) points out that piloting with a well-matched sample can also be extremely useful for foreshadowing potential dangers, ethical concerns or questions that may require more sensitive handling and delivery.

Bahn (2012) recommends that training on risk assessment be included in professional development training for research staff and students. Other important strategies include a call-in system when fieldworkers arrive at their data collection location and immediately afterwards, which means that each fieldworker should have a phone and be reimbursed for any use of that phone in the course of fieldwork duties. It may also be appropriate to consider sending fieldworkers out into the field in pairs. When working with vulnerable participants and children, it is important to consider the possibility of false allegations being made against fieldworkers and thus to limit a fieldworker's own vulnerability by having a protocol about not working alone and unobserved with a child or vulnerable person. Regular de-briefing sessions with the research supervisor and/or a research buddy will help to protect a fieldworker against the risk of becoming desensitized and will also increase the bond between the fieldworker and the supervisory team, meaning that fieldworkers are more likely to also share a sense of ownership and personal investment in the data.

Conclusion

Research studies published in peer-reviewed journals are less inclined to describe the recruitment, training or support of fieldworkers. This is despite the significant responsibilities that fieldworkers may have in terms of engaging with participants, gathering data and conducting the fieldwork in an ethical manner. The purpose of this chapter was to focus on some of the key issues relating to fieldwork, particularly in relation to the recruitment and training of fieldworkers, the potential for fieldwork behaviour to influence participants' responses and the practicalities involved in doing work in the field. In conclusion, the authors emphasize the need for researchers to reflect on the fieldwork process in order to support and promote high quality data collection and integrity.

References

Adams, S.A. *et al.* (2005) 'The effect of social desirability and social approval on self-reports of physical activity', *American Journal of Epidemiology*, 161(4), pp. 389–398.

Alexander, L. & Richman, K. (2008) 'Ethical dilemmas in evaluations using indigenous research workers', *American Journal of Evaluation*, 29(1), pp. 73–85.

Babbie, E. (1990) *Survey research methods.* 2nd edn. Belmont, CA: Wadsworth Publishing.

Bahn, S. (2012) 'Keeping academic field researchers safe: Ethical safeguards', *Journal of Academic Ethics*, 10(2), pp. 83–91.

Bahn, S. & Weatherill, P. (2013) 'Qualitative social research: A risky business when it comes to collecting "sensitive" data', *Qualitative Research*, 13, pp. 19–35.

Barker, J. & Weller, S. (2003) '"Never work with children?" The geography of methodological issues in research with children', *Qualitative Research*, 3, pp. 207–227.

Belousov, K. *et al.* (2007) 'Any port in a storm: Fieldwork difficulties in dangerous and crisis-ridden settings', *Qualitative Research*, 7(2), pp. 155–175.

Bernard, R.H. (2006) *Research methods in anthropology: Qualitative and quantitative approaches.* Lanham, MD: AltaMira.

Bjørkhaug, I., Perdersen, J. & Bøås, M. (2007) *Evaluation of the report 'Living conditions among people with activity limitations in Zambia'*. Oslo, Norway: Norwegian Federation of Organizations of Disabled People.

Bloor, M., Fincham, B. & Sampson, H. (2010) 'Unprepared for the worst: risks of harm for qualitative researchers', *Methodological Innovations Online*, 5(1), pp. 45–55.

Corbin, J. & Morse, J.M. (2003) 'The unstructured interactive interview: Issues of reciprocity and risks when dealing with sensitive topics', *Qualitative Inquiry*, 9(3), pp. 335–354.

Corsaro, W. (2005) *The sociology of childhood*. Thousand Oaks, CA: Pine Forge Press.

Crowne, D.P. & Marlowe, D. (1960) 'A new scale of social desirability independent of psychopathology', *Journal of Consulting Psychology*, 24, pp. 349–354.

Crutzen, R. & Goritz, A.S. (2010) 'Social desirability and self-reported health risk behaviors in web-based research: Three longitudinal studies', *BMC Public Health*, 10, p. 720.

Davis, C.G., Thake, J. & Vilhena, N. (2010) 'Social desirability biases in self-reported alcohol consumption and harms', *Addict Behavior*, 35(4), pp. 302–311.

Department of Children and Youth Affairs (2011) *Children first: National guidelines for the protection and welfare of children*. Dublin: Government Publications.

Dickson-Swift, V., James, E.L. & Kippen, S. (2005) 'Do university ethics committees adequately protect public health researchers?' *Australia and New Zealand Journal of Public Health*, 29(6), pp. 576–579.

Ebrahim, H.B. & Muthukrishna, N. (2005) 'Research with under fours: Some sense making moves', *Journal of Education*, 35, pp. 79–102.

Fisher, R.J. (1993) 'Social desirability bias and the validity of indirect questioning', *Journal of Consumer Research*, 20, pp. 303–315.

Fowler, F.J. (2002) *Survey research methods: Fundamental principles of clinical reasoning & research*. Thousand Oaks, CA: SAGE.

Goldstein, D.M. (2014) *Qualitative research in dangerous places: Becoming an "ethnographer" of violence and personal safety*. Social Science Research Council Working Papers. Available from www.ssrc.org/pages/qualitative-research-in-dangerous-places-becoming-an-ethnographer-of-violence-and-personal-safety/.

Green, L. & Baxen, J. (2002) 'The selection and training of fieldworkers in educational research: A Western Cape inquiry', *South African Journal of Education*, 22(4), pp. 319–325.

Gregory, K.E.& Radovinsky, L.(2012) 'Research strategies that result in optimal data collection from the patient medical record', *Applied Nursing Research*, 25(2), pp. 108–116.

Grosh, M. & Glewwe, P. (eds) (2000) *Designing household survey questionnaires for developing countries: Lessons from 15 years of the living standards measurement study*. Washington, DC: The World Bank.

Guinn, C.H. *et al.* (2010) 'Fourth-grade children's dietary recall accuracy for energy intake at school meals differs by social desirability and body mass index percentile in a study concerning retention interval', *Journal of Health Psychology*, 15(4), pp. 505–514.

Guinn, C.H. *et al.* (2008) 'Intrusions in children's dietary recalls: The roles of BMI, sex, race, interview protocol, and social desirability', *Obesity*, 16(9), pp. 2169–2174.

Hebert, J. R. *et al.* (2008) 'Social desirability trait influences on self-reported dietary measures among diverse participants in a multicenter multiple risk factor trial', *The Journal of Nutrition*, 138(1), pp. 226S–234S.

Hopkins, A. (2005) *Safety, culture and risk: The organisational causes of disasters*. Sydney: CCH Australia Ltd.

Hubbard, G., Backett-Milburn, K. & Kemmer, D. (2001) 'Working with emotion: issues for the researcher in fieldwork and teamwork', *International Journal of Social Research Methodology*, 4(2), pp. 119–137.

Jensen, P.S., Hoagwood, K. & Trickett, E.J. (1999) 'Ivory towers or earthen trenches? Community collaborations to foster "real world" research', *Applied Developmental Science*, 3, pp. 206–212.

Kitto, S.C., Chesters, J. & Grbich, C. (2008) Quality in qualitative research, *Medical Journal of Australia*, 188(4), pp. 243–246.

Kreuter, F., Presser, S. & Tourangeau, R. (2008) 'Social desirability bias in CATI, IVR, and web surveys: The effects of mode and question sensitivity', *Public Opinion Quarterly*, 72(5), pp. 847–865.

Lee, R.M. (1995) *Dangerous fieldwork*. Thousand Oaks, CA: SAGE.

Marshall, C. & Rossman, G.B. (1995) *Designing qualitative research*. Thousand Oaks, CA: SAGE.

Mitchell, W. & Irvine, A. (2008) 'I'm okay, you're okay? Reflections on the well-being and ethical requirements of researchers and research participants in conducting qualitative fieldwork interviews', *International Journal of Qualitative Methods*, 7(4), pp. 31–44.

Morrow, V. & Richards, M.P.M. (1996) 'The ethics of social research with children: An overview', *Children and Society*, 10, pp. 90–105.

Murphy, T. & Guerin, S. (2012) *How are our families? Report*. Dublin: Tallaght West Childhood Development Initiative.

Paterson, B.L., Gregory, D. & Thorne, S. (1999) 'A protocol for researcher Safety', *Qualitative Health Research*, 9(2), pp. 259–269.

Peterson, J. (2000) 'Sheer foolishness: Shifting definitions of danger in conducting and teaching ethnographic field research', in Lee-Treweek, G. & Linkogle, S. (eds) *Dangerous fieldwork: Risk and ethics in social research*. London: Routledge, pp. 181–196.

Sampson, H. (2004) 'Navigating the waves: the usefulness of a pilot in qualitative research', *Qualitative Research*, 4(3), pp. 383–402.

Sampson, H. & Thomas, M. (2003) 'Lone researchers at sea: Gender, risk and responsibility', *Qualitative Research*, 3, pp. 165–189.

Smith, J.A. (2008) *Qualitative psychology: A practical guide to research methods*. London: SAGE.

Sluka, J. (1990) 'Participant observation in violent social contexts', *Human Organization*, 49, pp. 114–126.

Tinson, J. (2009) *Conducting research with children and adolescents*. Oxford, UK: Goodfellow Publishers.

Tolbert, G.D. (2005) 'Residual risk reduction', *Professional Safety*, 50(11), pp. 25–33.

Tourangeau, R. & Yan, T. (2007) 'Sensitive questions in surveys', *Psychological Bulletin*, 133(5), pp. 859–883.

True, G., Alexander, L. & Richman, K. (2011) 'Misbehaviors of front-line research personnel and the integrity of community-based research', *Journal of Empirical Research on Human Research Ethics*, 6, pp. 3–12.

Üstun, T.B. *et al.* (2003) 'The world health surveys', in Murray, C.J.L. & Evans, D.B. (eds) *Health systems performance assessment: Debates, measures and empiricism*. Geneva: World Health Organization, pp. 797–808.

van de Mortel, T.F. (2009) 'Development of a questionnaire to assess health care students' hand hygiene knowledge, beliefs and practices', *Australian Journal of Advanced Nursing*, 26, pp. 9–16.

van Griensven, F. *et al.* (2006) 'Palmtop-assisted self-interviewing for the collection of sensitive behavioral data: randomized trial with drug use urine testing', *American Journal of Epidemiology*, 163(3), pp. 271–278.

Waller, T. & Bitou, A. (2011) 'Research with children: Three challenges for participatory research in early childhood', *European Early Childhood Education Research Journal*, 19, pp. 5–20.

Warming, H. (2005) 'Participant observation: A way to learn about children's perspectives', in Clarke, A., Kjørholt, A.T. & Moss, P. *Beyond listening: Children's perspectives on early childhood services.* Bristol: Policy Press, pp. 51–70.

8 Evaluating complex community change initiatives: Credible evidence is what counts

Morgan O'Brien and Sinead McGilloway

Introduction

The context for this chapter is the relatively recent growth in the prominence of large-scale area-based or community change initiatives (CCIs) which seek to implement strategic and comprehensive responses to the conditions and systems that contribute to and sustain poor outcomes at a community level. These initiatives, also commonly described as 'complex community initiatives' or 'comprehensive community initiatives' (see Kelly, 2010) or area-based initiatives (ABIs), are targeted, 'place-based' collaborative change efforts, which focus on specific areas and target populations rather than individuals. They aim to promote positive changes in individuals, families and communities by developing a variety of ways to improve identified outcomes, service provision and conditions in a targeted community; they place a particular emphasis on building community-level capacity and broader forms of systems change.

Arguably, given the scale and complexity of CCIs, more creative approaches to evaluation should be considered, but there are challenges involved therein. For example, the complexity, size and scope of these initiatives render it difficult, if not impossible, to isolate simple causal relationships which can be measured and tested using quantitative methods. Moreover, the environment within which they are implemented is often constantly changing, which presents challenges in terms of attempting to take into account all of the factors that might influence outcomes. Therefore, evaluations of CCIs and ABIs require a strong focus on documenting and analysing the 'how and why' of the programme (Saunders et al., 2005), especially as they evolve over time. We will return to this point later in the chapter.

New frameworks for conducting evaluations, which may be collectively described as 'theory-based approaches', offer useful alternatives for evaluators and programme stakeholders to explore and understand the implementation and perceived effectiveness of such programmes/initiatives. Specifically, this chapter describes the use of and challenges involved in theory-based evaluation approaches to area-based programmes and strategies and, in particular, CCIs. The discussion is contextualized, in part, with reference to an exemplar which involved an evaluation of an area-based strategy or CCI based in the Republic of Ireland called *youngballymun*, an initiative aimed at improving educational and wellbeing outcomes for disadvantaged children, young people and families. We argue that evaluations of complex initiatives such as *youngballymun* should focus mainly on data which provide a rich description of planning and implementation activities and allow for an in-depth analysis of multiple activities and processes of change (Connell & Kubisch, 1998; Kelly, 2010).

Characteristics of community change initiatives

CCIs can be broadly understood as a means of tackling multiple forms of deprivation (at a local or area-based level) in ways that recognize the nature of entrenched social problems in terms of their environmental origins, their complexity and their interrelatedness (O'Connor, 1995). The rationale for the development and implementation of these kinds of initiatives lies in recognizing the ways in which locality and neighbourhood can significantly shape access to opportunities and demarcate forms of disadvantage and inequality.

CCIs are tailored to meet community needs and circumstances which, as might be expected, can lead to differences in their emphasis and focus. For example, Kubisch (2010) identifies two categories of CCI. The first is classified as 'physical revitalization and economic development', which focuses on the built environment mainly through the construction of affordable housing and the promotion of commercial and economic development. The second type of CCI identified by Kubisch (2010) focuses on 'human development and social services' and may target a range of issues, including education, health and family wellbeing.

However, whilst CCIs may vary in terms of their specific aims and objectives, they all include, at their core, 'community building' and 'comprehensiveness'/a 'comprehensive lens' (Kubisch, 2010). According to Kubisch (2010, p. 12), the emphasis on the 'community building' process relates to the "linking of the people and place dimension of this work" through engagement with the local community and promoting ownership of that process. The development of a 'comprehensive lens' refers to the way in which CCIs work across multiple levels, including individual, community, organizations and systems. This allows such initiatives to address specific outcomes, whilst also retaining an understanding of how community issues can be implicated in wider social and economic structures. Thus, CCIs tend to adopt an approach that: (a) operates according to community development/community-building principles; (b) emphasizes local engagement and community capacity building; and (c) implements strategies that seek to activate public and private/philanthropic funding in pursuit of longer-term systemic change (see Kubisch et al., 1995).

youngballymun as a community change initiatives

youngballymun was established in 2007 with joint funding from The Atlantic Philanthropies (AP) and the former Office of the Minister for Children and

Youth Affairs (OMCYA). This initiative comprises five child-, youth- and family-centred service strategies designed to improve learning and wellbeing outcomes for all children and young people (and their families) in Ballymun. Ballymun is an area in North Dublin which has long been characterized by high levels of disadvantage. Traditionally, the area has had a significant involvement in community development processes and a long history of local community activism (Boyle, 2005). Ballymun has also received significant levels of government funding to support policies and programmes aimed at improving the provision of local community services and their attendant outcomes. For example, prior to the development of *youngballymun*, the area had received considerable funding which was administered through an organization called Ballymun Regeneration, which was established in 1997. The aim of this funding was to improve the built environment through the construction of affordable housing and the development of commercial and economic potential.

The *youngballymun* initiative may be conceptualized as a CCI in that it attempts to address problems holistically to effect change at multiple levels (individual, family, community). It strives to achieve its goals by means of integrating activities and strategies across a range of systems/sectors, whilst also engaging the wider community in order to, ultimately, achieve sustainable forms of systemic change. The initiative was funded as part of the broader Prevention and Early Intervention Programme (PEIP) which was designed to provide innovative programmes to foster better outcomes for children, young people and families living in disadvantaged areas (Department of the Taoiseach, 2006). This programme targeted three geographic areas in Dublin where there was evidence of high levels of need – Ballymun, Tallaght West and Darndale. The overarching aim of the PEIP was to support the development, implementation and evaluation of strategies for children at a local level as identified by the statutory, voluntary and community agencies operating within the relevant areas. The PEIP has since been replaced by the new Area-Based Child Poverty (ABC) programme, which is a prevention and early intervention initiative that has adopted an area-based approach, across thirteen sites, to improve outcomes for children who are at risk of or experiencing poverty.

The PEIP strategy and its successor both recognize the importance of early intervention and prevention and the utilization of evidence-based and evidence-informed practices and services in reducing or removing the risks associated with disadvantage and promoting positive outcomes for children and their families. This reflects a considerable body of international evidence (as discussed throughout this text) which shows that socioeconomic disadvantage (amongst other things) is a major factor in constraining early life development and that early childhood intervention is key to addressing a range of negative longer-term outcomes; these include poor educational attainment, early school leaving, mental health problems, social difficulties, substance abuse, as well as poor employment prospects and an increased reliance on welfare and social care systems (e.g. Collishaw et al., 2004; Fergusson, Horwood & Ridder, 2005; Colman et al., 2009).

youngballymun may be viewed as the second type of CCI described above, in that it focuses on 'human development and social services' and targets a range of issues, including education, health and family wellbeing. Indeed, the general principles associated with CCIs are evident within the programme of work and strategic goals of *youngballymun*. In particular, the local initiative actively pursued a prevention and early intervention model in line with the strategic goals of the PEIP. Its overarching aim was (and is) to ensure that statutory and community/voluntary services work more effectively to improve the learning and wellbeing outcomes of children and young people (and their families) living in Ballymun. This was, at least in part, to be realized through the establishment of five service strategies that target identified needs across the life cycle of a child in three main areas: literacy and language, health and development and mental health.

These five service strategies were located within an overarching comprehensive change strategy which sought, from its inception, to work with existing statutory agencies and community-based organizations in order to bring about lasting change in service provision and practice and encourage the adoption of evidence-based, outcomes-focused approaches. Specifically, the five services and the overall strategy reflected a commitment by *youngballymun* from the outset to: (1) promote innovative evidence-based programmes and evidence-informed practice; (2) encourage collaborative and integrated practices/ways of working through multi-stakeholder engagement; (3) build capacity in families, amongst practitioners and within services; (4) promote an 'outcomes-focused' culture of service provision; and (5) ultimately foster lasting systemic change (i.e. change across multiple levels and systems). These five goals formed the framework for the evaluation that is discussed later in this chapter.

The five *youngballymun* services were designed to be delivered across the child–youth lifespan and to create learning opportunities that enabled services and institutions to change and enhance their effectiveness. As such, the initiative reflects the comprehensive nature of CCIs more generally. At a strategy level, it advocates redirecting the emphasis on investment of resources to earlier in the life of a child, using evidence-informed practice. This is based on the premise that existing systems and services intervene too late in the lifespan of children in disadvantaged communities to impact significantly on their outcomes. Therefore, *youngballymun* sought, from the outset, to be transformative across a number of levels, including individuals, families, services, institutions and policies. Thus, its wide range of activities, at the time of the study, included direct service delivery, capacity building, awareness raising, developing an impetus and infrastructure for change and providing asset-building opportunities.

Evaluating community change initiatives: Challenges for evaluators

CCIs focus on implementing 'best practices' and 'evidence-based programmes' in areas such as workforce development, child and family services and education, in order to improve the wellbeing of children and families and to catalyse transformation at a community level (Kubisch et al., 2010). This emphasis on developing and introducing new programmes based on robust evidence has led to an increased interest in identifying appropriate and meaningful ways of evaluating such initiatives.

Evaluation research plays a key role in assessing the (perceived and actual) effectiveness, utility and acceptability of CCIs, how they operate and how they attempt to effect change at both an individual and community level, as well as wider forms of strategic change. In 2009 the *youngballymun* programme directors commissioned an overarching process evaluation (as well as separate evaluations of each if its five services) to assess the overall impact of the initiative and to appraise its role, in particular, in fostering meaningful and lasting forms of systemic change in services for local children, young people and families. As indicated earlier, this evaluation (in which both authors were involved as part of a larger team) provides a useful exemplar (and context) for this chapter (McGilloway et al., 2013).

Discussions of CCIs typically emphasize the central importance of evaluation as a means to fully understand and articulate how such programmes operate and attempt to cultivate change at both a community and strategic level. However, the characteristics of CCIs – and in particular their wide-ranging and multipartite nature and their focus on multiple, diverse outcomes – present significant challenges for evaluators seeking to produce relevant and credible evidence on their effectiveness and impact. As Coote, Allen and Woodhead (2004, p. 48) suggest, such initiatives are "hard to evaluate because of their size and the speed with which they are being rolled out, and because they are trying to address multiple problems within shifting political environments".

As discussed, CCIs such as *youngballymun* are inherently complex interventions. Firstly, they are horizontally complex insofar as they implement and attempt to achieve synergy across numerous strands of work within multiple sectors and systems simultaneously (Kelly, 2010). Secondly, they are vertically complex in that they seek to realize change at many levels (i.e. individual, family, organization, community and system levels) and are predicated on the notion that there is interaction and influence between these levels (Kubisch et al., 2010). Thus, such initiatives propose to generate outcomes which are often difficult to measure and can change over time. Contextual issues add another layer of complexity and, in particular, the macroeconomic climate, which can have a direct bearing on the success of a CCI, and over which such an initiative may have little influence. This level of complexity can present significant challenges for developing appropriate evaluative approaches, over and above the practical and methodological difficulties of any successful evaluation.

There is often a mismatch between the timeframe of a CCI and the programme of work involved in its evaluation. For instance, the kinds of change that CCIs such as *youngballymun* are expected to produce in a given community usually take longer than the lifespan of an initiative. Therefore, long-term follow-up is ideally required to determine whether the anticipated outcomes actually materialize and whether any changes that occur in the short term are sustained (Craig et al., 2008). Thus, it is unlikely that traditional outcome measures will show much change during the lifetime of the evaluation, even though such change might be expected in the long run. Consequently, it is important that evaluators of CCIs distinguish short-term from intermediate and longer-term outcomes. This is compounded by the fact that CCIs usually have a lengthy start-up phase, as implementation is typically slow.

In the US, the planning and design of CCIs is more likely to be integrated with the development of evaluation strategies in parallel. However, more commonly in the UK and Ireland, while evaluations are usually a requirement of publicly funded initiatives, they often commence after the programme or intervention is established (see Sullivan, Barnes & Matka, 2002). This approach means that evaluations often take place after an initiative has had time to 'bed down' and become properly established and well-functioning. Specifically, in the context of the evaluation of *youngballymun*, the study was initiated after the initiative had been designed and implementation had begun. Therefore, while the potential for the evaluation to inform aspects of *youngballymun*'s strategic plan or programme of work was limited, the study as a whole was able to contribute to and inform the ongoing evolution of the initiative as it progressed.

Another challenge for evaluators is the need to capture elements of the initiative that go beyond narrow programmatic outcomes. Fundamental to CCIs is the belief that a synergy will be achieved by providing a comprehensive range of interventions/services. Evaluations that focus only on discrete programme components and/or programmatic outcomes may ignore, or fail to detect, the effects of their interaction, whilst tracking and measuring such synergy is also difficult.

Evaluators also face the challenge of addressing the mismatch between the demands for evaluations of CCIs that are both rigorous and useful to policy-makers and programme developers and traditional evaluation methods which may not allow such utility. For example, evidence-based medicine applies a hierarchical approach to evaluations whereby levels of evidence are defined by the study design and execution. Accordingly, designs have been variously graded by their potential to eliminate bias. The highest level of evidence is based on research involving randomized controlled trials (RCTs) with usually large numbers of participants, whilst the lowest level relates to descriptive studies (e.g. case series) and expert opinion (Sanson-Fisher et al., 2007). The concept of 'levels of evidence' has been widely promoted to inform guidelines and recommendations for clinical practice, and has been increasingly applied to other areas of evidence-based decision making, including social and educational programmes.

However, CCIs do not fit the accepted paradigms of programme evaluation that emphasize the use of experimental or quasi-experimental approaches and particularly RCTs, an issue noted in several chapters in this text. For example, these initiatives are designed to target *all* individuals in a given geographical area and, therefore, there is a high level of community saturation, which means that randomly allocating individuals to 'treatment' and 'control' groups for the purposes of ascertaining a counterfactual (i.e. what would have happened in the absence of the initiative) is often not possible or ethically desirable. An alternative might be to look at the situation before and after such an initiative is implemented in a given community, or to use comparison communities. However, communities are complex and dynamic, with frequent changes in target outcomes, even in the absence of any intentional interventions (Kelly, 2010). Therefore, assessments of the situation before the initiative or in comparison communities may not provide reliable counterfactuals, as they may not accurately represent what the community would have looked like in the absence of the initiative.

While there is considerable support for the notion of using research evidence to continually improve efficiency and effectiveness, there is a lack of consensus about what constitutes sound evidence for decision-making. It has been increasingly acknowledged that the 'hierarchy of evidence' favours interventions most amenable to certain types of study design, particularly those with a medical rather than a public health or social focus, and interventions targeting individuals rather than populations. This growing critique of the usefulness of the 'hierarchy of evidence' framework as an appropriate model for working with people who receive community-based interventions has led to the development of evaluation approaches that seek to provide alternative ways of understanding their effectiveness (Julnes & Rog, 2009). This is especially so in the case of CCIs.

Theory-based evaluations of community change initiatives

The evaluation challenges presented by large-scale, complex, community-based programmes and interventions have led to a growing emphasis in relatively recent years on strategies that allow evaluators to address the 'theory' of how such programmes work (or are intended to work) and to take account of the context in which they operate (Hills, 2004). Stame (2004) argued that the growing emphasis on theory-based approaches to evaluation was driven by a desire to open the 'black box' within which the processes or pathways that lead from cause to effect are hidden. A key advantage, according to Weiss (1997), of adopting a theory-based approach, is that it can be used to identify the aspects of an initiative that lead to outcomes by focusing on the link between the processes and the causal mechanisms underpinning an initiative. This approach has emerged as particularly relevant and useful in the evaluation of programmes of work, such as CCIs, which seek to address multiple forms of change across varying levels (e.g. individual, community, systems, etc.). The role of theory-based evaluation is central to the evaluation of CCIs as considered in this chapter.

In general, theory-based evaluation (TBE) is a broad term that has also been variously referred to as 'theory-driven' evaluation, 'program theory', 'intervention theory' and 'theory of change' (see Funnell & Rogers, 2011; Rogers, 2007). Whilst there is some variation amongst these, a general principle of this approach to evaluation involves articulating the 'theory' of an initiative or programme by identifying the set of guiding assumptions that underpin its work (Funnell & Rogers, 2011). As Birckmayer and Weiss (2000, p. 408) summarize:

> It is an approach to evaluation that requires surfacing the assumptions on which the program is based in considerable detail: what activities are being conducted, what effect each particular activity will have, what the program does next, what the expected response is, what happens next, and so on, to the expected outcomes.

Chen's (1990) *Theory-Driven Evaluation* provided a significant impetus to the progression of theory-based evaluation in the early to mid-1990s, which was subsequently developed by the Aspen Round Table in two collections detailing the use of theory-based approaches, and particularly the application of theory of change (ToC), in the evaluation of CCIs (Connell et al., 1995; Fulbright-Anderson, Kubisch & Connell, 1998). Such an approach offers ways of moving past input–output description and, in simple terms, provides evaluative evidence based on how a programme does or does not work. Mason and Barnes (2007) indicate that while ToC approaches have been applied with considerable variation, they are consistent with the broader principles of theory-based evaluation in seeking to identify the set of assumptions (or 'theories') about what should happen in order for specific forms of change to occur.

Weiss (1995) defines a ToC as being fundamentally a theory of how and why an initiative works. A ToC evaluation identifies the causal pathways intended to lead to particular outcomes rather than focusing on identifying and measuring the outcomes of an initiative. In practice, this involves delineating the micro-steps, or causal chain, that leads from inputs to outcomes and allows the evaluators to explore how and why the initiative is intended to work. The evaluators can then use the results of this process to demonstrate where the steps in the causal chain produce, or fail to produce, intended results.

However, there has been considerable debate about what exactly is meant by 'theory' and, in turn, debate about how theory-based evaluations are conducted. Weiss (1997) draws a distinction between 'implementation theory', which identifies what is needed to translate objectives into service delivery and programme operation, and 'programme theory', which, she argues, refers to the hypothesized causal links between mechanisms of an intervention and their anticipated outcomes. Evaluators using a theory-based approach, Weiss (1997) argues, often tend to focus on implementation rather than programme theory, and emphasize sets of activities that are then linked to intermediate outcomes without necessarily demonstrating the causal mechanisms that are intended to be produced by an initiative. Programme theory, on the other hand, focuses on the mechanisms that mediate the relationship between activities and outcomes (e.g. the response generated by the provision of training, such as giving recipients greater knowledge or confidence).

It has been suggested that evaluations that focus only on implementation theory are limited in that they test the assumption that if an initiative is carried out with fidelity, the intended outcomes will occur – without necessarily explaining why or how a particular initiative works. More recently, Rogers (2007) suggests that organizations and evaluators who claim to utilize programme theory are often, instead, very much focused on implementation theory and the attendant (and frequent) use of logic models. She argues that whilst logic models provide a useful starting point:

> These simple diagrams fall short of the conceptual summary involved in a programmatic theory because they do not examine the causal mechanisms involved in programs and policies ... and do not show the different complementary or alternate causal strands in achieving the outcomes.
>
> (Rogers, 2007, p. 64).

Alternatively, the use of programme theory allows evaluators to address the mechanisms that link programme inputs to particular outcomes and to describe responses to particular activities, rather than just the activities themselves.

Likewise, Leuww and Donaldson (2015) distinguish between differing conceptualizations of implementation and programme theory, which they describe as 'theories of policy makers, stakeholders and evaluators'. They argue that cumulatively these "in one way or another build on the assumptions that underlie programs" (Leuww & Donaldson, 2015, p. 469). The same authors identify a second type of theory relevant to evaluation, which they describe as: "scientific theories capable of contextualizing and explaining the consequences of policies, programs and evaluators' actions". This theory is derived from existing research evidence, particularly in the context of social, behavioural or institutional science, which helps to explain how policies are developed and implemented, or to explore how an initiative operates in its social and institutional context. According to Leuww and Donaldson (2015, p. 472), theory-based evaluations should ideally incorporate both of these theoretical approaches because those based on academic or scientific ideas can also provide "crucial insights about mechanisms and contexts underlying policies and programs, including evaluation interventions".

Stern et al. (2012, p. 25) also indicate how the term 'theory', in the context of evaluation research, is used in "various" and "inconsistent" ways. They distinguish between two main and interrelated trends within theory-based approaches to evaluation (see also Stame, 2004). The first is articulated as 'process oriented', which views programmes as involving causal pathways that lead to particular outcomes. This approach, evident in ToC evaluations (as outlined above), allows evaluators to identify the causal pathways that are anticipated to lead to intended goals and under what conditions. The second is to focus on 'mechanisms', which are seen as conditioning factors that make a programme work. This is most usually associated with realistic evaluation (RE) approaches as developed by Pawson and Tilley (1997), who argue that this shifts the emphasis "from asking whether a programme works to understanding what it is about a programme that makes it work" (p. 67). Specifically, Pawson and Tilley (1997) argue that the context of an initiative or programme influences the mechanisms that lead to particular outcomes, and that by exploring the interaction of CMOs (that is, context, mechanisms and outcomes), evaluators can uncover how and why an initiative or programme has the potential to effect change. For Pawson and Tilley, it is not the initiatives themselves that produce change, but the mechanisms often implicit in them and the way in which they are activated for individuals and groups in particular contexts.

Blamey and Mackenzie (2007) suggest that ToC and RE approaches, whilst different in a number of ways, can be used in an integrated manner to address different elements in an evaluation. They argue that both approaches seek to identify aspects of implementation and programme theory (see also Stame, 2004). They further state that ToC approaches typically focus on large-scale, complex, community-based interventions, whilst the examples of RE as discussed by Pawson and Tilley (1997) tend toward more focused programmes or individual policy domains, such as prisoner education programmes or CCTV interventions for crime prevention. However, they assert that "many policy programmes lend themselves to the explicit testing of a dual Theories of Change/Realistic Evaluation model" (Blamey & MacKenzie, p. 452), such that ToC is suited to clarifying implementation theory whilst RE is used to discern 'micro-level' elements of programme theory.

More recently, Stern et al. (2012) observed that evaluators will often integrate and combine these two elements in practice. For instance, both Carroll et al. (2005) and Secker et al. (2005) outline cases where the design and implementation of evaluations of health promotion initiatives involved a combination of RE/ToC approaches. Indeed, Secker et al. (2005, p. 394) suggest that a "theories of change approach [...] fits well with the realistic evaluation design, facilitating a more in-depth exploration of the relationship between contexts, mechanisms and outcomes". Arguably, therefore, the integration of ToC and RE allows for a description of what happened and why, but also addresses issues of causality, and why and how the initiative produced positive or negative outcomes under particular circumstances.

Applying a theory-based approach to the evaluation of *youngballymun*

The principal aim of the evaluation of the *youngballymun* initiative was to appraise its overall impact during an approximate three-year period, particularly with a view to informing its development and evolution into the second phase of its ten-year strategy. The evaluation focused on the activities and processes initiated as part of the overall programme/strategy that influenced its implementation and development and were conceptualized within the context of TBE approaches. In simple terms, the evaluation set out to ascertain:

- What worked in the development, implementation and evolution of *youngballymun* and under what conditions/circumstances?
- What did not work and why?
- What key lessons emerged at the mid-way stage of the initiative?

As outlined above, the application of theory-based evaluation in real world research has progressed in varying and, at times, contrasting ways. In particular, the understanding of theory and how it might be best understood, described and used in providing credible evaluation results is still a subject of extensive discussion and debate. In the context of implementing a theory-based approach to the evaluation of *youngballymun*, we attempted to identify some lessons from the literature in order to develop our evaluation design, questions and methods. An approach informed by Blamey and MacKenzie's (2007) integrated ToC/RE approach was identified as a particularly relevant and useful means of identifying and articulating: (1) the intended causal pathways and assumptions underlining *youngballymun*'s programme of work (that is, implementation theory); and (2) the transformation process itself and why/how particular activities or interventions produce, or do not produce, intended and desired results (that is, programme theory).

As noted above, logic models are often viewed as lacking sophistication and being overly descriptive of programmatic activities rather than identifying causal mechanisms – as defined in both articulations of programme theory within ToC and RE. However, they have become increasingly used as iterations of theory in the evaluations of CCIs (Stern, 2004). Stern (2004, pp. 31–32), whilst acknowledging the limitations of logic models due to "their lack of explanatory power and a-theoretical nature", concludes that such applications of logic models may benefit from a synthesis with theory-based approaches.

In the context of the evaluation of *youngballymun*, it was identified, through an initial documentary analysis and a series of in-depth interviews, that the logic model of the initiative was based on a meaningful and legitimate process of design and development involving a wide range of relevant stakeholders at community, sectoral and institutional/policy levels. As with many CCIs, *youngballymun* was perceived to be based on an identifiable set of values and principles, and, importantly, on a logic model, which articulated its core mission and objectives. This provided a useful starting point and context within which to develop and address relevant themes and issues relating to the building of 'theory', with specific reference to the values and objectives of the initiative. This emphasis was reflected in the planning, design and method of the evaluation. In particular, the logic model provided an initial context within which to examine and define the key assumptions underpinning *youngballymun*. As such, this logic model offered a relevant and useful initial form of implementation theory, which provided a detailed description of how *youngballymun* intended to produce specific short-term, medium-term and long-term outcomes.

This approach allowed the evaluation team to develop a series of more specific evaluation questions that informed the research design and guided subsequent data collection and analysis. These questions incorporated activities, processes and structures that fell within four overarching themes/issues that had been identified – in discussion with the *youngballymun* Research Steering Group – as central to the development and activities of the initiative and therefore as crucial to our evaluation. These included: (1) the early design and development of the *youngballymun* initiative, including institution building and organizational capacity (e.g. organizational structures that set goals, encouraged participation and provided effective leadership and guidance); (2) engagement, partnership working and collaboration (e.g. that allowed for the exchange of information, development and achievement of shared goals and the building of trust and promotion of interagency working); (3) capacity building (e.g. that encompassed selection, training and coaching to improve skills and which encouraged best practice and innovation for practitioners and services); and (4) systems change and longer-term integration of services and practice (e.g. whereby the initiative demonstrated that it was sensitive to addressing multi-level change by working towards the establishment of sustainable change across different systems such as local services, administrative layers, policy). A fifth theme, 'value for money', was addressed in a separate economic sub-study commissioned as part of the evaluation and which was conducted in parallel (see Lawlor & McGilloway, 2012).

Each of these themes was examined and explored within a broader implementation science framework which allowed us to consider how *youngballymun* fared with respect to each theme at different stages of implementation, including its planning and design/strategic development, initial and full implementation, innovation/integration and sustainability (Fixsen et al., 2009). Each thematic domain also represented relevant intended causal pathways and assumptions which were identified, both explicitly and implicitly, as central to *youngballymun*'s programme of work. The next stage of the evaluation was to develop an understanding of these causal mechanisms or the programme theory elements (Weiss, 1997). The evaluation sought, in particular, to assess how these activities and their contexts might be hypothesized to activate mechanisms that lead to change.

For example, a key goal of the *youngballymun* initiative, at the time of our study, was to build capacity and, in many ways, its success or otherwise relied/relies largely on the impact and overall effectiveness of its capacity building endeavours. Despite this, the explicit role of capacity building in improving learning and wellbeing outcomes in Ballymun and, in particular, the means and mechanisms by which capacity could be developed, were not clearly articulated within the *youngballymun* logic model. However, the *youngballymun* Implementation Plan described the role of capacity building as "strengthening the ability of individuals, groups, and organizations to build the skills, systems and structures they need to better achieve their objectives" (youngballymun, 2010, p. 39). More specifically, capacity building was understood to be critical to achieving "enhanced educational and wellbeing outcomes for children and young people in Ballymun" (ibid. p. 26).

This demonstrated that, while there was a clear assumption that varying forms of capacity building activities were hypothesized to produce intended programmatic and strategic outcomes, the key mechanisms that such activities might be anticipated to trigger were not clearly articulated; in other words, what was it about the forms of capacity building being undertaken that led to these outcomes and in what contexts? Accordingly, the evaluation identified and utilized both underlying stakeholder theories of capacity building along with appropriate models from the relevant social science literature (e.g. Chaskin, 2001) to identify how forms of capacity building activities at varying levels, including, for example, community-based practitioners, might operate to produce change.

For example, existing theory highlights the importance of mentoring, coaching and modelling as particularly important in helping to generate new individual capacities and, crucially, in facilitating the translation of these into changed practices. Current evidence also suggests that the implementation of new skills (and intervention programmes) requires varying degrees of behaviour change amongst practitioners (Fixsen & Blase, 2009). Supporting 'on the job' behaviour change through mentoring, coaching and modelling provides practitioners with opportunities to practise and apply skills, whilst also offering appropriate encouragement and advice (Fixsen et al., 2009). Indeed, 'on the job' supports have been identified as key 'implementation drivers' (or enablers) in ensuring implementation and implementation fidelity and, when added to the kinds of training seen here, can lead to substantial improvements in practitioner skills and knowledge (Fixsen & Blase, 2009).

These aspects were then used as a means of exploring and analysing the numerous capacity building activities of *youngballymun*, as well as identifying key facilitative and inhibitive factors underpinning those activities. For example, we hypothesized that where *youngballymun* sought to build practitioner capacity in working with children, young people and families, such activities should be built on: (a) fostering positive relationships between *youngballymun* staff and community-based practitioners who were seen as responding to needs; (b) implementing activities tailored to meet practitioners' capacity/work role; (c) ensuring that skills and practices are compatible with existing goals; and (d) using ongoing support (e.g. mentoring, coaching, modelling) to translate activities into action. These were essentially used as a means to identify and 'test' particular context/mechanism configurations, whereby it was identified that where these elements were present, they facilitated the introduction and embedding of new, evidence-informed practices into existing services.

This approach was applied across all of the thematic domains outlined above to identify ways in which the work/activities of *youngballymun* could be understood and how these were leading to intended outcomes (if at all). In this way, the emergent findings from the evaluation helped to inform the ongoing development of the initiative by providing credible evidence on what aspects of the programme were working well (or not), and, more importantly, the 'why' and the 'how' of such activities and processes and the key lessons for potential replicability elsewhere.

For example, the evaluation findings indicate, amongst other things, that *youngballymun* pursued numerous and diverse capacity building activities across individual, organizational/service and environmental levels (McGilloway et al., 2013). These aimed to help the initiative gain the trust of the community and led to important improvements in awareness, engagement, practitioner skill/knowledge development and the implementation of evidence-based and evidence-informed practices. As part of this process, *youngballymun* established organizational structures to facilitate the ongoing inclusion of local organizations during its implementation, which helped to build positive working relationships and establish shared goals. At the same time, however, capacity building became more difficult to pursue in instances where service providers felt their voices were not heard or included.

Thus, capacity building activities were most successful when they: were tailored to be accessible; met the needs of local organizations; and were rolled out in a phased manner in order to ensure that individual organizations were able to incrementally implement practices in a systematic and sustainable basis that fitted with existing work roles and capacity. For example, within the early childcare and primary education sectors, *youngballymun* staff focused their capacity building efforts on meeting the needs of childcare facilities and primary schools, as well as allowing time for consolidation and appropriate reflection. Where these elements were present, it was found that services benefited from access to practical resources and relevant forms of staff training/mentoring which, in turn, contributed to improved practitioner confidence, knowledge and skills.

Conclusion

This chapter explored some of the challenges of evaluating CCIs and how the features and principles of theory-based evaluation might be applied to better understand and explore the processes initiated and developed by CCIs; an exemplar from the Republic of Ireland was used to contextualize, in part, this discussion. While there are differing and at times competing conceptualizations of what 'theory' might relate to in the context of TBE, arguably such debates are useful in providing a set of guiding principles on how these kinds of evaluations may be conducted. As Coryn et al. (2011, p. 203) state, TBE is animated by two key elements: "Conceptually, theory-driven evaluations should explicate a program theory or model. Empirically, theory-driven evaluations seek to investigate how programs cause intended or observed outcomes".

Our overall evaluation approach illustrates the merits of using a combined ToC and RE approach to provide important insights into the various stages of implementation (and processes and mechanisms therein) of a CCI, including, in particular, service design/strategic development, engagement, collaboration and partnership working, capacity building and integration/systems change. All of these were identified as thematic domains highly relevant to the local initiative and, therefore, key to the aims and objectives of the evaluation. Further details can be found in our evaluation report (available at www.youngballymun.org), which also identified some key messages/lessons for other CCIs, as well as a number of challenges which emerged (and were for the most part resolved) during the different stages of implementation.

Acknowledgements

We would like to extend our thanks to: The Atlantic Philanthropies who funded the evaluation of *youngballymun*; all those who kindly participated in and facilitated the research; including all *youngballymun* staff and all members of the evaluation research team, including Dr Grainne Hickey, Ms Yvonne Leckey, Professor Michael Donnelly, Professor Maurice Devlin and Professor Elliot Stern. We are also grateful to Gemma Cox for her contribution to the development of this chapter.

References

Birckmayer, J.D. & Weiss, C.H. (2000) 'Theory based evaluation in practice: What do we learn?' *Evaluation Review*, 24(4), pp. 407–431.

Blamey, A. & Mackenzie, M. (2007) 'Theories of change and realistic evaluation. Peas in a pod or apples and oranges?' *Evaluation*, 13(4), pp. 439–455.

Boyle, M. (2005) 'Sartre's circular dialectic and the empires of abstract space: A history of space and place in Ballymun, Dublin', *Annals of the Association of the American Geographers*, 95, pp. 181–201.

Carroll, M. *et al.* (2005) 'A realistic/theory of change approach to the evaluation of health promotion in small- and medium-sized enterprises in Sandwell', *Social Policy & Society* 4(4), pp. 393–401.

Chaskin, R.J. (2001) 'Building community capacity: A definitional framework and case studies from a comprehensive community initiative', *Urban Affairs Review*, 36, pp. 291–324.

Chen, H.T. (1990) *Theory driven evaluations.* London: SAGE.

Collishaw, S. *et al.* (2004) 'Time trends in adolescent mental health', *Journal of Child Psychology and Psychiatry*, 45, pp. 1350–1362.

Colman, I. *et al.* (2009) 'Outcomes of conduct problems in adolescence: 40 year follow-up of a national cohort', *British Medical Journal*, 338, pp. 208–211.

Connell, J. & Kubisch, A.C. (1998) 'Applying a theory of change approach to evaluating comprehensive community initiatives', in Fulbright-Anderson, K., Kubisch, A.C. & Connell, J. (eds) *New Approaches to Evaluating Community Initiatives, Vol 2.* Washington, DC: Aspen Institute, pp. 15–44.

Connell, J.P. *et al.* (eds) (1995) *New approaches to evaluating community initiatives: Concepts, methods, and contexts.* Washington, DC: The Aspen Institute.

Coote, A., Allen, J. & Woodhead, D. (2004) *Finding out what works: Building knowledge about complex, community-based initiatives.* London: King's Fund.

Coryn, C. *et al.* (2011) 'A systematic review of theory-driven evaluation practice from 1990 to 2009', *American Journal of Evaluation*, 32(2), pp. 199–226.

Craig, P. *et al.* (2008) 'Developing and evaluating complex interventions: The new Medical Research Council guidance', *BMJ*, 337, pp. 979–983.

Department of the Taoiseach (2006) *Towards 2016: Ten-year framework social partnership agreement 2006–2015.* Dublin: Stationery Office.

Fergusson, D.M., Horwood, L.J. & Ridder, E.M. (2005) 'Show me the child at seven: The consequences of conduct problems in childhood for psychosocial functioning in adulthood', *Journal of Child Psychology and Psychiatry*, 46, pp. 837–849.

Fixsen, D.L. & Blase, K.A. (2009) *Implementation: The missing link between research and practice. NIRN implementation brief #1.* Chapel Hill, NC: The University of North Carolina, FPG: National Implementation Research Network.

Fixsen, D.L. *et al.* (2009) 'Core implementation components', *Research on Social Work Practice*, 19, pp. 531–540.

Fulbright-Anderson, K., Kubisch, A.C. & Connell, J.P. (eds) (1998) *New approaches to evaluating community initiatives, Vol 2.* Washington, DC: The Aspen Institute.

Funnell, S. & Rogers, P. (2011) *Purposeful program theory: Effective use of theories of change and logic models.* San Francisco, CA: Jossey-Bass/Wiley.

Hills, D. (2004) *Evaluation of community-level interventions for health improvement: A review of experience in the UK.* London: Health Development Agency.

Julnes, G., & Rog, D. (2009) 'Evaluation methods for producing actionable evidence: Contextual influences on adequacy and appropriateness of method choice', in Donaldson, S.I., Christie, C.A. & Mark, M.M. (eds) *What counts as credible evidence in applied research and evaluation practice?* Thousand Oaks, CA: SAGE, pp. 96–132.

Kelly, T. (2010) 'Five simple rules for evaluating complex community initiatives', *Community Investments*, 22, pp. 19–36.

Kubisch, A.C. (2010) 'Recent history of community change efforts in the United States', in Kubisch, A.C. *et al.* (eds) *Voices from the field III: Lessons and challenges from two decades of community change efforts.* Washington, DC: Aspen Institute, pp. 8–14.

Kubisch, A.C. *et al.* (2010) 'Community change initiatives from 1990–2010: Accomplishments and implications for future work', *Community Investments*, 22, pp. 8–12.

Kubisch, A.C. *et al.* (1995) 'Introduction', in Connell, J.P. *et al.* (eds) *New approaches to evaluating community initiatives: Concepts, methods, and contexts.* Washington, DC: The Aspen Institute, pp. 1–22.

Lawlor, E. & McGilloway, S. (2012) *An economic appraisal of the youngballymun initiative.* London: Just Economics.

Leuww, F.L. & Donaldson, S.I. (2015) 'Theory in evaluation: Reducing confusion and encouraging debate', *Evaluation*, 21(4), pp. 467–480.

Mason, P. & Barnes, M. (2007) 'Constructing theories of change: Methods and sources', *Evaluation*, 13(2), pp. 151–170.

McGilloway, S. *et al.* (2013) *A process evaluation of youngballymun.* Dublin: Youngballymun.

O'Connor, A. (1995) 'Evaluating comprehensive community initiatives: A view from history', in Connell, J.P. *et al.* (eds) (1995) *New approaches to evaluating community initiatives: Concepts, methods, and contexts.* Washington, DC: The Aspen Institute, pp. 23–64.

Pawson, R. & Tilley, N. (1997) *Realistic evaluation.* London: SAGE.

Rogers, P. (2007) 'Theory-based evaluation: Reflections ten years on', *New Directions for Evaluation*, 114, pp. 63–67.

Sanson-Fisher, R. *et al.* (2007) 'Limitations of the randomised control trial in evaluating population-based health interventions', *American Journal of Preventive Medicine*, 33(2), pp. 155–161.

Saunders, R.P., Evans, M.H. and Joshi, P. (2005) 'Developing a process evaluation plan for assessing health promotion program implementation: A how-to guide', *Health Promotion Practice*, 6(2), pp. 134–147.

Secker, J. *et al.* (2005) 'Theories of change: What works in improving health in mid-life?' *Health Education Research: Theory & Practice*, 20(4), pp. 392–401.

Stame, N. (2004) 'Theory based evaluation and types of complexity', *Evaluation*, 10(1), pp. 58–76.

Stern, E. (2004) 'Philosophies and types of evaluation research', in Descy, P. & Tessaring, M. (eds) *The foundations of evaluation and impact research. Third report on vocational training research in Europe: Background report.* Luxembourg: Office for Official Publications of the European Communities (Cedefop Reference series, 58), pp. 11–50.

Stern, E. *et al.* (2012) *Broadening the range and design of methods for impact evaluations.* Working Paper 38. London: Department for International Development.

Sullivan, H., Barnes, M. & Matka, E. (2002) 'Building collaborative capacity through "Theories of Change": Early lessons from the evaluation of health action zones in England', *Evaluation*, 8(2), pp. 205–226.

Weiss, C. (1997) 'Theory based evaluation: Past, present and future', *New Directions for Evaluation*, 76, pp. 41–55.

Weiss, C. (1995) 'Nothing as practical as good theory: Exploring theory-based evaluation in complex community initiatives for children and families', in Connell, J.P. *et al.* (eds) *New approaches to evaluating community initiatives: Concepts, methods, and contexts.* Washington, DC: Aspen Institute, pp. 65–92.

youngballymun (2010) *youngballymun implementation plan.* Dublin: youngballymun.

9 Community-based dissemination of research findings

Gemma Kiernan and Marian Quinn

Introduction

An integral element of undertaking community-based research and evaluation in national and international settings is ensuring that research findings are actively disseminated to key stakeholders. This communication is central to the responsive approach to research discussed in Chapter 2. The premise of this chapter is that undertaking research in a community setting is not a purely academic or 'ivory tower' process, but one which should impact on communities and those who live in them, enhance understanding of the lives of children and families through informing community leaders, support effective, evidence-informed decision-making and contribute to the use of proven intervention strategies in community environments. The chapter will consider exemplary dissemination of research findings to key stakeholders within community settings and highlight those factors that can support or hinder this process. The chapter which follows (Chapter 10) considers dissemination at the broadest level, which typically focuses on the policy context.

Successful dissemination is a key part of the research process, and indeed effective feedback loops are central to maintaining the engagement and motivation of stakeholders and optimizing the likelihood that research findings can inform policy, practice and resource allocations (McDavitt et al., 2016). Dissemination has relevance for maximizing the possibility that research is positioned to result in improved outcomes for communities in areas such as education, health and wellbeing (DCYA, 2011). In the past, many guides for students and new researchers failed to mention dissemination strategies as a core aspect of planning and completing research (Kane, 1993; Pawson & Tilley, 1997). Indeed, it is only in recent years that funding for research has included a requirement for and the resources to enable effective knowledge transfer and exchange (see Chapter 10). There is increasing recognition of the importance of translating and communicating research to maximize impact and improve outcomes for children and families and a growing emphasis on the value of knowledge transfer and exchange as part of the research process. Therefore, it is both necessary and timely to consider the often complex dissemination process and to support its careful consideration as an integral aspect of the research process.

Despite the increase in community-based research in recent years, there is a limited but growing body of knowledge on effective dissemination of research to those considered to be primary audiences, the immediate stakeholders and those that may be secondary audiences – those working in the wider context (Cohen et al., 2015). Depending on the nature of the research, community-based stakeholders (i.e. those living and working in the community, the primary audience) may include those directly and indirectly involved in the delivery or receipt of services being evaluated, such as managers, frontline staff, residents including parents and children and other related professionals. These are the focus of this chapter. Other stakeholders (the secondary audience) who are not based in the community must also be considered in terms of dissemination, as their expertise, role or influence is potentially significant. These include other communities, academics, policymakers and influencers such as advocacy groups, politicians, professional organizations and the media. These multi-faceted and diverse groups require targeted, tailored engagement, with messaging that maximizes the likelihood of the research learning being further disseminated (see Cohen et al., 2015). These secondary stakeholders are discussed in Chapter 10.

This chapter starts with an examination of models and strategies for effective and meaningful engagement with primary stakeholders in relation to community dissemination of research findings. Following this, the challenges involved in disseminating research findings into community settings will be considered, and examples from a community-based programme in a disadvantaged area in Dublin, Ireland will be used as illustration (see www.twcdi.ie). Then a summary of the key factors to facilitate successful dissemination will be identified. Finally, the chapter will close with consideration of how commitment to successful dissemination can enrich the quality and effectiveness of community-based research.

Models and strategies for community-based dissemination

It has been suggested that dissemination may be best regarded as a complex process. Drawing on the Push-Pull infrastructure model developed by the Robert Wood Johnson Foundation (Orleans, 2003), Kerner, Rimer and Emmons (2005) posit that there needs to be receptivity to the research findings (i.e. pull from community-based stakeholders) and at the same time a concerted effort to help disseminate and implement the findings (i.e. push from researchers and/or their funders). For dissemination to be successful, there must be an emphasis on increasing pull or desire for the research and research findings from the community-based stakeholders and on improving the push from researchers.

The principles of community-based participatory research (forms of which are considered in other chapters in this text) are relevant to maximizing understanding of children's and families' lives within their communities. Bergold and Thomas (2012) define these as including: 'democratic' principles, or the need for a social and political context and a research commitment to enabling an equitable voice for all stakeholders, the creation of a 'safe space' in which participants can speak honestly and where diverse perspectives and contradictory opinions are welcomed and heard; consideration of who participates and how 'the community' is defined, with particular acknowledgement of those groups which have difficulty engaging and where tailored approaches may be required; and finally, the principle that stakeholders are involved in and have a level of control at every stage of the research. When community-based organizations are involved as full partners in research design, implementation and consideration of study findings, these organizations and the individuals within them are likely to 'pull', that is, be open to and eager for the research and demanding of research findings. In relation to dissemination, it is recommended that stakeholders should be involved in interpreting and applying the findings (Green & Mercer, 2001). There is evidence to show that partnering with community members as co-researchers can make a critical contribution to dissemination by conveying knowledge that is relevant and credible to communities (Genius, Willows, Nation & Jardine, 2015).

The number of and variation in stakeholders means that dissemination requires careful conceptualization and planning to be successful. It should by no means be assumed that there will be sectoral allegiances, whereby all residents, for example, have the same priorities, or that all professionals have a shared vision of what the community requires. Children, parents and professionals will often have quite different views on the priority needs in the community and how best to address these. Inevitably, there will be competing and at times contradictory perspectives which will inform the research itself as well as the mechanisms by which to disseminate the learning. Awareness of the power relationships at play, and how to develop trust in relationships, will be important if all stakeholders are to remain engaged (Christopher, Watts, McCormick & Young, 2008). While stakeholders should be consulted and involved in relation to the interpretation of findings prior to formal dissemination, there is not always a need for this to be an overly labour intensive process.

Researchers, for their part, must be conscious of the nature of the 'push' they give in relation to dissemination. Given that there are typically challenges associated with engaging community-based stakeholders, sensitivity, adaptability and indeed creativity are required in relation to the methods of disseminating the research (Genius, Willows, Nation & Jardine, 2015). For such innovation to be realized in dissemination, researchers must be encouraged and supported by funding agencies and peer review bodies and may require increased funding to enable dissemination efforts (Kerner et al., 2005). Commissioners of community research should be cognizant of this when allocating funding and agreeing timelines. Recognition of the resources and skills required to support these processes should underpin agreements between those funding and those undertaking such research.

In disseminating the findings from a longitudinal study examining the relationship between social network characteristics and health outcomes for black people living with HIV (Hoover et al., 2015), McDavitt et al. (2016)

developed a framework for community-based dissemination. This could provide a means through which to operationalize the 'push-pull' model and provides a series of overlapping phases, emphasizing the centrality of ongoing dialogue with the community and the development of trust between the researchers and community stakeholders. The phases are outlined in Box 9.1.

Box 9.1 Operationalizing push-pull factors in dissemination (McDavitt et al., 2016)

- Planning: Activities suggested include integrating community dissemination into the research aims, and utilizing existing structures for communication rather than developing new ones.
- Reaching out to community partners: It is suggested that this will be most effectively implemented by identifying a designated person to lead on communication, holding pre-meetings with gatekeepers and drawing on established relationships.
- Tailoring content for various audiences: The framework proposes that findings can be shared in terms of their research function, implications for policy or their practical application, and that the emphasis on each of these will depend on the audience.
- Sharing the findings: Methods to maximize dialogue and support interactive engagement are discussed, including the use of personal anecdotes, and researchers being receptive to criticism.
- Follow-up: The importance of researchers planning for and being open to ongoing dialogue is stressed with examples including meetings, conference calls, and so on, with a focus on implications, implementation and possible further collaboration.

An example of balanced engagement in the dissemination process with community stakeholders comes from the Tallaght West Childhood Development Initiative (CDI) in West Dublin, Ireland (see www.twcdi.ie). The CDI is a community response to the needs of children and families in a disadvantaged community in Dublin and it has designed and supported the implementation of a range of services for this population. As part of this, CDI commissioned seven service evaluations which were subsequently disseminated to stakeholders in the community and nationally. In order to prepare for and facilitate effective dissemination, a reflection group process was initiated by CDI for each of its evaluations, in which each independent research team individually presented an overview of research methodology, findings and conclusions to groups of up to 25 key stakeholders. The groups included representatives from residents and parents, school principals, health services, local authorities, police and the voluntary sector. Minimizing technical language and presenting the conclusions in relation to 'What does this mean for this community and wider afield?' enabled meaningful engagement and deepened understanding amongst those who had participated in the research. This process not only increased the knowledge and ownership of the research within the community, but gave research teams a process by which to 'sanity check' their findings, ensure the context was appropriately reflected, and consider the balance of conclusions. As is evident from this example, a major advantage of this process of balanced and meaningful engagement with stakeholders in terms of dissemination lies in the fact that it has the potential to improve the external validity of research and to maximize the applicability of research findings to community settings. Through doing so, it increases the likelihood of local 'pull', which might increase the likelihood of impact from the research.

Whilst the above framework may provide a practical and useful guide for approaching community-based dissemination, challenges will inevitably occur. These will now be considered.

Negotiating challenges

In a systematic review, Chen, Diaz, Lucas and Rosenthal (2010) evaluated 101 articles reporting on studies using the community-based participatory research approach to characterize dissemination for research results beyond scientific publication. They found dissemination of findings to community participants and the general public to be largely occurring but marked by myriad challenges. The pertinent challenges they and other researchers have noted include negotiating challenging findings; receptivity of community members to findings; complexity in conveying findings in an accessible and relevant way which recognizes the reality of children's and families' lives; problems in the relationship between the researchers and the community; and resourcing and time constraints (Christopher, Watts, McCormick & Young, 2008; Makhoul, Nakkash, Harpham & Qutteina, 2013; Chen, Diaz, Lucas & Rosenthal, 2010). Each of these challenges is considered in more depth below, including strategies to navigate them.

Negotiating challenging findings

In community-based research, challenging findings may include a range of outcomes. The evidence might suggest that a key stakeholder did not engage in the intervention effectively or that the intervention was ineffective in achieving the intended outcomes despite significant resources being invested. There may be a concern that improvements in outcomes as a result of the intervention will result in reduced funding, or evidence that one intervention or service is outperforming another might create local tensions and competition. Researchers and community-based stakeholders need to decide in advance how challenging findings are to be documented and released. Indeed, Travers and Flicker (2004) suggest that the ethical review process at the front end of every community research project should require a statement of built-in mechanisms for dealing with 'negative' findings. Having such a statement may help in that it can serve as a protocol for how to write up and convey challenging findings. It is also important that researchers preserve the integrity of findings whilst being sensitive to the potential implications that conveying challenging findings may have on people's lives and working relationships. Development of such a statement should include consideration of the following:

- Who owns the data? Who is responsible for disseminating the findings?
- What are the potentially problematic findings and how might these be managed?
- How can different views on the dissemination of the findings be managed?
- Commitment to being transparent, independent of the results.
- Effective engagement of all stakeholders in considering the conclusions from the research.
- Strategies for use when significant difficulties arise, including support from other parties.

Community receptivity

There are of course other challenges relating to the dissemination of research findings, even in the event that the conclusions are positive. The receptivity of community members to the research process, including the dissemination of findings, may be affected by the physical, structural and social conditions of the community context. For example, in a study of a youth mental health intervention built on researcher–community partnership in a Palestinian refugee camp in Beirut, Lebanon (Makhoul, Nakkash, Harpham & Qutteina, 2013), multiple factors compromised effective community engagement in the research process. These included political restrictions, poverty, instability and uncertainty and parental concern considerations. Most of these factors were beyond the researchers' control, but they require attention and in relation to dissemination they may mean that children and families are not always in a receptive space to consider research findings and implications. Makhoul, Nakkash, Harpham and Qutteina (2013) suggest the need for pilot grants that help assess the extent of the complexity in community conditions and identify aspects that may help or hinder the research process. This model of piloting needs to be extended to include dissemination to allow researchers to explore the process of sharing the findings.

Dealing with complexity

In relation to the complexity of conveying findings in an accessible way, researchers need to be sensitive to the language used, and include comprehensive explanations as well as making helpful recommendations for going forward. Ensuring that language and concepts used are not alienating or confusing for people, whilst also avoiding patronizing the community, is important (Chen, Diaz, Lucas & Rosenthal, 2010). This is often best managed through a partnership between the research team and the commissioner, or local community organizations with whom residents have an ongoing relationship. Involving children in dissemination brings additional considerations in terms of developmentally appropriate language and communication methods. Again, balancing the integrity of the messages with a focus on ensuring meaningful dialogue is important. As noted above, a partnership with local organizations will support this process and offer parents and service providers reassurance about its validity.

Resources and time constraints

Resources and demands on time can be a major factor in determining the quality of dissemination and whether it gets any attention at all. With broad-based dissemination, where the goal is to use research findings to encourage action towards improving the lives of children and families, there is a need to resource a range of innovative and meaningful activities to ensure knowledge transfer. This can be costly and needs to be built into funding requests from the outset. In terms of demands on time, Chen, Diaz, Lucas and Rosenthal (2010) highlight how people, especially those with lower incomes, are typically very busy with priorities other than engaging with the dissemination process.

In disseminating the findings from seven independent evaluations, the Tallaght West Childhood Development Initiative (CDI), referenced above, utilized some innovative mechanisms to engage parents and children to ensure that the findings were accessible and relevant. A family day was held in a community sports hall, with various local champions and politicians calling in throughout the day. Games were developed for each evaluation, whereby the successful completion of a game provided the answer to a research related question. For example, throw the hoop over the ring which you think indicates the percentage by which children in the ‘Doodle Den’ intervention improved their reading. As well as the CDI staff, a team of over thirty local volunteers supported the day, talking to people about the research and promoting the services in the area. All families received a ‘goodie bag’ with healthy snacks, vouchers from the local swimming pool and information about services and how to use them. Encouraging attendance on the day was a lengthy and hugely resource intensive piece of work, drawing on the volunteers and local schools and services, as well as having events and activities to attract families. An ice cream van was at the event all day, and everyone who completed a game got a ticket for an ice cream. A local singer who had been a finalist on *The Voice of Ireland* ended the afternoon. Over 300 families participated in the day, many of them staying for several hours talking to people connected with CDI.

There was no formal evaluation of the event, or attempt to assess subsequent outcomes, but on reflection it did provide an opportunity for the staff to re-engage with volunteers and parents with whom there had been little contact for some time. It also gave the organization direct contact with new families who had been participating in services and in the weeks following the event, a number of parents phoned the office looking for advice on specific issues, generally relating to accessing specialist services. It can be implied from this that participants saw CDI as a source of support and local knowledge. Informal feedback subsequent to the event was that it had been enjoyed by the families who attended but that many only heard about the family day after it took place. This latter feedback was frustrating for those involved given the time and resources assigned to publicizing the event, but perhaps not surprising given the size of the community, the diversity of families, and the inherent difficulties in communicating effectively in this environment.

Dealing with difficult relationships

A different type of challenge can occur in the dissemination process if there is a relationship breakdown between the researchers and the community-based stakeholders. There are organizational differences between research staff and those in community-based organizations and this, coupled with differing priorities, agendas and work practices can often place a strain on the relationship between the two groups. Establishing effective communication strategies that include regular updates and meetings from the outset, transparent expectations and processes for troubleshooting and managing tensions will prove invaluable. Agreeing these at the start of the partnership will offset future difficulties. These issues are discussed in detail in Chapter 3 of this text.

Related to differing perspectives, a further challenge in dissemination can arise if stakeholders have different expectations regarding the sequencing of dissemination (Chen Diaz, Lucas & Rosenthal, 2010). In some instances, for example, researchers may want to publish findings according to timelines more suited to their academic institution requirements and before they are disseminated and implemented in the community. The commissioner of the research may wish to present findings at a practice-based forum in advance of the evaluation report being finalized or peer reviewed articles being published, and funders may be anxious to use interim findings to inform future funding decisions. Clarity regarding ownership of the data will inform how these decisions get made, as will a mutual understanding of the relevant perspectives and contexts within which the partners work. However, Chen et al. (2010) give examples of a more deep-seated approach whereby communities have established research centres that are owned and funded by communities themselves, independent of academic partners and consequently of their timelines for publication.

A case study of managing dissemination

As a case study of how to manage challenges in disseminating findings, we present the example of research commissioned by the aforementioned CDI to develop an evidence-informed programme to support pro-social behaviour in nine- to 10-year-olds (O'Hare, Kerr, Biggart & Connolly, 2012). This manualized programme was evaluated over three years, using a randomized controlled trial (RCT), whilst service delivery was commissioned to an established voluntary service working in the area. The rolling cohort design of the RCT found that after three years, of the 21 outcomes measured, there had been no impact on 16. There was a negative impact on three of the measures, and two were moving in a positive direction, but did not reach statistical significance. These results were not only disappointing, given the level of investment and the confidence in the evidence basis of the programme; they were unexpected and upsetting for stakeholders, as the process aspects of the evaluation had been largely very positive. Children, parents and teachers spoke warmly of the programme, and whilst not universally positive, feedback indicated an overall sense that the intervention was having benefit. The results of the RCT were such that it was agreed between CDI and the evaluation team that the manualized programme must cease delivery with immediate effect. Consideration of those stakeholders with whom to communicate this decision identified the groups reported in Box 9.2.

Box 9.2 Groups identified as stakeholders

- Participating children
- Parents of children in the intervention group
- Parents of children in the control group
- Facilitators delivering the programme
- Managers of the commissioned service
- School teachers and principals
- Other professionals who may have referred children to the service, e.g. educational psychology
- CDI governance structures, including funders

There was a recognition throughout this process that maintaining the trust and support of these stakeholders was central to CDI, not only due to ongoing work and the centrality of continued partnership,[1] but because participating in and supporting an RCT had been a leap of faith for many individuals and organizations – an uncomfortable and ethically challenging approach that tested values, relationships and priorities. In this context, clear and transparent communication was a minimum expectation. The open and trusting relationship between the commissioner (CDI) and the research team played no small part in enabling this approach. Having a common philosophy and confidence in the integrity underpinning this inevitably difficult engagement was critical.

Having identified the various stakeholders, careful consideration was given to the sequence of engagement and information sharing. The following approaches were taken in this chronological order:

- Service Managers: The two managers of the service provider responsible for delivery of the programme were invited to meet with CDI and the evaluation team, having explained in a telephone conversation that there were disappointing results from the evaluation. There was then a series of meetings with the managers agreeing the various next steps of communication, and the managers were involved throughout each of these.
- Frontline Facilitators: The facilitators who directly delivered the programme to the children were initially informed of the research findings by their managers. A meeting then took place with CDI and the evaluation team at which the findings were discussed in greater detail.
- School Principals: A letter for the school principals was drafted between CDI, the evaluation team and the service manager. This was then hand delivered to each of the seven participating schools by the CEO of CDI, and where possible, the contents of the letter were discussed face to face.
- Parents: The parents/guardians of all children who had ever received the intervention were written to, with the support of the schools and service delivery organization. This letter, agreed using the same approach as for the letter for school principals, set out three bullet points outlining the key findings from the evaluation in simple language. Parents were also invited to attend an open meeting to discuss the evaluation, which was attended by the evaluation team, service managers, some facilitators and CDI. Sign language was provided for one parent to facilitate participation.
- Children: It was agreed that children would continue to receive a service until the end of the academic year, as would have been expected. Elements of the original programme approach were retained, through agreement between the service provider and evaluation team, in order to maintain consistency for the children, in particular in relation to behaviour management. Other elements of delivery to the children were drawn from a well-established programme used by the service provider.

Throughout the process, which was conducted within ten working days of the first meeting, a range of responses was identified with a high degree of consistency across the various stakeholders. These included denial ("I don't believe it"), guilt ("What did we do wrong?"), anger ("Why didn't you tell us sooner?") and finally acceptance ("That's really disappointing"). In short, the stakeholders were observed to have moved through the stages of bereavement akin to those outlined in models of grief (e.g. Kübler-Ross, 2005).

In addition to the above engagement with key stakeholders, CDI undertook several precautionary steps in order to prepare for the possibility that the 'bad news' was brought to local media or politicians, or indeed that any of the stakeholders saw litigation as an appropriate response to the negative findings. Legal advice was sought in finalizing all correspondence, a draft press release was prepared for circulation in the event that local media drew attention to the fact that a service had been proven to be ineffective, and a letter to local politicians was drafted. None of these was ultimately required, and it was CDI's belief that the care, attention and detail given to this time consuming, emotional and difficult process enabled even the most avid champions of the programme to accept the findings. This was enabled by the fact that the relationship between the research team and the commissioner was such that there was a shared principle of respecting the community stakeholders and the need to maintain relationships for the future. This reiterates findings by researchers such as McDavitt et al. (2016) and Burke et al. (2013) about the importance of communication and trust between the researchers, commissioners and community stakeholders during the dissemination process.

Key factors to support effective community-based dissemination

In our review of the models and strategies for community-based dissemination and the associated challenges, which drew on the international literature and case studies, numerous approaches have been highlighted that support successful dissemination.

Of central importance is the need for a respectful working relationship between researchers and community-based stakeholders. Building a mutually respectful and trusting relationship takes a significant investment of time and requires negotiation, but it pays dividends when it comes to dissemination (McDavitt et al. 2016). It requires compatibility between the research organization(s), the community organization(s) and local representatives, with each understanding one another's structure and culture. If these are in place, the benefit is easier dissemination with the minimum of tensions. Indeed, studies reporting on and evaluating the diffusion and dissemination of research findings in communities have shown that taking time to understand each other's perspectives enabled more meaningful recommendations to be made regarding the implications of research findings for practice innovations (e.g. Slater, Finnegan & Madigan, 2005).

Effective management of community-based research projects plays a vital role in contributing to successful dissemination. For example, a research project steering group consisting of residents and key local service providers may act as 'first port of call' to read drafts and advise on the most appropriate and useful dissemination strategies. Ideally, this group will have been engaged from the outset of the research process, and have had a role in agreeing its focus and methodology. It also necessitates that there are agreed roles and responsibilities and clear lines of communication. Clarity regarding ownership of research and the research findings, including intellectual property and data, should be addressed. This issue is discussed in greater detail in Chapter 3 of this publication. Dissemination must be planned and intentional for it to be successful and occur in a systematic manner. There needs to be an agreed infrastructure and process for dissemination of research findings with clarity of expectations between researchers and the community-based stakeholders regarding deliverables and timelines. Without this information, there is a danger that the research and research findings will only be diffused by researchers through more 'academic' means, including conference presentations and journal articles (Kerner et al., 2005).

As already alluded to above, careful consideration needs to be given to the methods of dissemination within community-based settings. Ensuring that dissemination processes are accessible to the various audiences is important in terms of the language used, physical locations and the means of inviting participation. Cognizance of the local context should inform the identification of appropriate incentives (Chen, Diaz, Lucas & Rosenthal, 2010), and an openness and capacity for creative methods of dissemination will support this process. This may require tailored training for researchers in order to upskill them in community engagement processes around dissemination. Opportunities for stakeholder feedback on research processes and dissemination are also central to establishing and maintaining buy-in.

Conclusion

Sharing findings from community-based research is a complex process, without clear guidelines on how best to go about it, nor consistent, effective structures to facilitate it. As with all communication processes, the interests, perspectives and motivation of the target audience should be considered in order to inform the methods, timing and appropriate media to share key messages. Creativity, investment of time, energy and resources, and insights based on effective working relationships will all contribute to the planning for effective dissemination. At the core of the strategies which can facilitate effective dissemination is the relationship between the researcher, the commissioner and the community. Working arrangements based on respect, recognition of difference and a commitment to working collaboratively are fundamental to ensuring that research undertaken in community settings is meaningful, helpful and a positive experience for all involved. Recognizing the power relationships which are inherent in even the most collaborative processes between disadvantaged communities and researchers is a necessary precursor to establishing these working methods. At the same time, the principles of good governance must apply and so risk assessment and measures to minimize potential difficulties are equally central.

Exemplary dissemination reaps many benefits. Principally, it has the potential to enrich the overall quality of community-based research and improve the validity of findings. However, effective engagement at this stage of the research process can have more far reaching impacts as well, such as collaborating to create a more research literate and analytical community; demonstrating a more democratic and inclusive process which may positively impact on the tensions and mistrust which can arise between communities, academics and service providers; increasing local understanding and ownership of both the process and the conclusions; and consequently contributing to the likelihood of translating such findings into action to help community members, specifically children and families.

Acknowledgements

The authors would like to thank the Department of Children and Youth Affairs in Ireland, and The Atlantic Philanthropies who supported much of the work referenced above.

Note

1 For the purposes of this chapter, the term 'commissioner' is used to refer to the organization that sought and funded the research.

References

Bergold, J. & Thomas, S. (2012) 'Participatory research methods: a methodological approach in motion', *Forum Qualitative Sozialforschung/Forum: Qualitative Social Research*, 13(1), Art. 30. Available from http://nbn-resolving.de/urn:nbn:de:0114-fqs1201302.

Burke, J. G., Hess, S., Hoffmann, K., Guizzetti, L., Loy, E., Gielen, A., Bailey, M., Walnoha, A., Barbee, G. & Yonas, M. (2013) 'Translating community based participatory research principles into practice', *Progress in Community Health Partnerships: Research, Education, and Action*, 7(2), pp. 115–122.

Chen, P.G., Diaz, N., Lucas, G.& Rosenthal, M.S. (2010) 'Dissemination of results in community based participatory research', *American Journal of Preventive Medicine*, 39(4), pp. 372–378.

Christopher, S., Watts, V., McCormick, A.K.H.G. & Young, S. (2008) 'Building and maintaining trust in a community based participatory research partnership', *American Journal of Public Health*, 98(8), pp. 1398–1406.

Cohen, E.L. *et al.* (2015) 'Designing for dissemination: Lessons in message design from "1-2-3Pap"', *Health Communication*, 30(2), pp. 196–207. doi:10.1080/10410236. 2014.974130

DCYA (2011) *National strategy for research and data on children's lives.* Dublin: Department of Children and Youth Affairs, pp. 2011–2016.

Genius, S.K., Willows, N., Nation, A.F. & Jardine, C.G. (2015) 'Partnering with indigenous student co-researchers: Improving research processes and outcomes', *International Journal of Circumpolar Health*, 74. doi:10.3402/ijch.v74.27838

Green, L.W. & Mercer, S.L. (2001) 'Can public health researchers and agencies reconcile the push from funding bodies and the pull from communities?' *American Journal of Public Health*, 91(12), pp. 1926–1929.

Hoover, M.A. *et al.* (2015) 'Do people know i'm poz?: Factors associated with knowledge of serostatus among HIV-positive African Americans' social network members', *AIDS and Behavior*, 20(1), pp. 137–146.

Kane, E. (1993) *Doing your own research.* New York, NY: Marion Boyers.

Kerner, J., Rimer, B. & Emmons, K. (2005) 'Introduction to the special section on dissemination: Dissemination research and research dissemination: How can we close the gap?' *Health Psychology*, 24(5), pp. 443–446.

Kübler-Ross, E. (2005) *On grief and grieving: Finding the meaning of grief through the five stages of loss.* New York, NY: Simon & Schuster Ltd.

Makhoul, J., Nakkash, R., Harpham, T. & Qutteina, Y. (2013) 'Community-based participatory research in complex settings: Clean mind-dirty hands', *Health Promotion International*, 29(3), pp. 510–517. doi:10.1093/heapro/dat049

McDavitt, B. et al. (2016) 'Dissemination as dialogue: Building trust and sharing research findings through community engagement', *Preventing Chronic Disease*, 13, pp. 1–7. doi:10.5888/ped13.150473

O'Hare, L., Kerr, K., Biggart, A., and Connolly, P. (2012) *Evaluation of the effectiveness of the Childhood Development Initiative's Mate-Tricks pro-social behaviour after-school programme.* Dublin: Childhood Development Initiative.

Orleans, C.T. (2003) 'The larger challenge of translation: An extraordinary opportunity for cancer control'. http://cancercontrol.cancer.gov/d4d/pdfs/challenge_translation.pdf

Pawson, R. and Tilley, N. (1997) *Realistic evaluation.* London: Sage.

Slater, J.S., Finnegan, J.R. Jr. & Madigan, S.D. (2005) 'Incorporation of a successful community-based mammography intervention: Dissemination beyond a community trial', *Health Psychology*, 24, pp. 463–469.

Travers, R. & Flicker, S. (2004) *Ethical issues in community based research.* Urban Health Community-Based Research Series Workshop. Wellesley, MA: Wellesley Institute.

10 Knowledge exchange: Informing policy and influencing change

Nóirín Hayes and Maresa Duignan

Introduction

Most researchers involved in applied social science would like to see their research having an impact on policy and practice. One of the best ways to achieve this is through making research findings available to a wide and varied audience. While many universities and higher education institutions have local mechanisms to support researchers in the dissemination of their findings and/or products, these links rarely involve direct connection between the research, policy and practitioner stakeholders into the "iron triangle" which Feldman (1999) has argued is essential for real research impact on policy.

How best to achieve impact from research has become a subject of study over the last decade, and the findings suggest that the task is a difficult one (Datta, 2012). Drawing on national and international experience, this chapter will consider the nature of knowledge exchange and the requirements necessary to enhance the impact of research findings on policy development and implementation. It will briefly review what impacts – direct and indirect – the increased importance being placed on academic research has had on policy formation, implementation and practice.

Building on the previous chapter, we explore the growth of a knowledge exchange culture and the role of knowledge brokering in policy developments from the joint authorial perspective of a research and a policy base in Ireland. We hope that the points raised will be valuable across different research disciplines, institutions and government departments.

Policy development

Traditionally, policy development has been characterized as a linear model, whereby policy is seen as a sequential process broken down into discrete elements. Despite the intuition of linearity, it is now understood that public policy development and implementation is driven and influenced by the interaction of complex social, political and economic forces. The last decade has seen a significant increase in investment by governments in real world community-based research initiatives. Such investment reflects the increased attention policy makers are giving to research evidence as a basis for policy development. Policy bodies seek evidence from the academic research community to guide future policy. "This is particularly the case with children, where significant changes in their growth, development and outcomes take place within a relatively short period" (Department of Children and Youth Affairs, 2011, p. 2). This is not easy to achieve, as the relationship between research evidence and its use in practice or by policymakers is far from straightforward and may be quite unpredictable.

For instance, national policy pertaining to children in Ireland has undergone a radical shift in both vision and implementation in the decades since 1990. The publication of the Irish Child Care Act of 1991, which effectively replaced the previously pertinent legislation, the 1908 Children's Act, marked the commencement of a series of policy developments which addressed the provision of services and supports for children. These are too numerous to detail in this chapter, but reflect a general shift in Irish policy attention to children driven by both national and international developments, including the ratification of the UN Convention on the Rights of the Child in 1992. Evidence of the significance of the national developments can be seen in the move from the appointment of a Junior Minister for Children in 2000 to the establishment of a National Children's Office and through to the current position with the formation of the Department of Children and Youth Affairs (DCYA) (Hayes, 2006; Duignan, 2011).

Many factors can be identified as having had an impact on the various policy actions described above, but often the impact is only seen retrospectively. For example, it was during this decade that the scandalous treatment of children at the hands of both the State and its agents over previous decades began to emerge and, as Richardson (1999, p. 181) claimed, "the current period in the development of childcare policy has been characterised by the implementation of new legislation and dominated by increasing public awareness of physical and sexual abuse as a major factor in Irish society".

As the above illustrates, different factors can work to move policy along. There are several barriers to influencing the direction of policy or practice and they reflect, among other things, the different cultures of the research, policy and practice environments. Lyall (2008) suggests that whilst the more traditional academic research may impact policy and practice, this impact is indirect and more long term, and the knowledge transfer/knowledge exchange literature emphasizes the non-linear, often incidental nature of such research impacts. Policymakers do not respond as academics, and require short, clear and timely pieces of work to inform the decision-making process, whereas for much research – particularly in the social sciences – research findings serve to raise new questions as well as answering those under research consideration.

In the wider context of the UN Convention on the Rights of the Child, the past two decades have witnessed a significant growth in Irish research activity relating to the lives and experiences of children in Ireland. This has been driven by the commitment of the National Children's Strategy (2000), which identified understanding children's lives as a key goal of the ten-year plan. Additionally, the State recognized the value and importance of policy development that is informed by rigorous research evidence, and to that end channelled funding into a number of key initiatives, including the National Children's Office (latterly subsumed into the DCYA), the Centre for Early Childhood Development and Education (2002–2008) and the Growing Up in Ireland national longitudinal study of children's lives (see www.esri.ie/growing-up-in-ireland/). During this time, philanthropic activity, which has always had a strong presence in supporting the delivery of service provision for children, has stimulated and supported the development of an indigenous research base through the establishment and support of large-scale projects such as the Prevention and Early Intervention Programme (PEIP) projects in Ireland (reported in several chapters in this text) alongside investment in capacity building in research. Retrospectively, these various factors contributed to a changed policy climate and witnessed a closer level of interaction between the traditionally disconnected domains of research, policy and practice. This feature, described in the literature as knowledge exchange, was supported by a range of factors, and it is these factors that are now discussed in the context of the literature through exploring how the essential elements of knowledge exchange processes can continue to be harnessed.

Knowledge exchange

When attention initially began to focus on the valuable potential of research in the development of policy, there was an emphasis on the need for knowledge transfer from researchers to policymakers. The limitations of the uni-directional model were quickly recognized, and the term was revised to 'knowledge exchange'. Knowledge exchange has been defined as the "interaction between decision makers and researchers that results in mutual learning through the process of planning, producing, disseminating and applying existing or new research in decision making" (Canadian Health Services Research Foundation [CHRSF], cited in Goldfeld, 2010, p. 2). They further suggest that whilst the first and primary objective of knowledge exchange is to support evidence-based decision-making, a corollary and arguably a condition of success in knowledge exchange is the promotion of mutual understanding between researchers and decision makers. The importance of knowledge exchange has also been recognized at a European level. From a European Commission perspective, funded projects have always been required to illustrate 'valorization' of the investment of resources in research and development. Valorization can be described as a process of exploiting project learning and outcomes (training products and processes, methodology, course materials, etc.) with a view to optimizing their value and impact in existing and new contexts (target groups, companies, sectors, training institutions and systems, etc.) (Moser & Zebra, 2011). To achieve this, however, takes more than simple partnership and, as Duignan (2011) has argued, can take time to develop and grow to the point of yielding the concrete policy and practice outcomes.

A factor in this temporal dimension to the impact of research on policy and practice is that greater insight into differences across professional cultures requires persistence and is time consuming. The establishment of a partnership approach to evidence-based decision-making at an early stage in the research/policy process is one approach to facilitating effective and efficient knowledge exchange. The idea of creating a partnership between policymakers and researchers would seem logical, and indeed in Ireland in the past two decades there has been an increase in such activity whereby the research questions are established in line with the direction/ambitions of national policymaking. However, as Lyall (2008) has noted, there is a tension here particularly for the research community, where close partnership with decision makers is often interpreted by researchers as constraining and limiting for research design, process and output. She argues that it is useful to examine the differences between academic research and policy research when aiming for collaborative engagement across both sectors. For instance, she notes that the purpose of research is understood differently; researchers see research as gathering "knowledge for understanding" while policymakers see it as "knowledge for action" (2008, p. 4). Researchers are not overtly political whereas policymakers argue that the political aspects of research cannot be ignored or suppressed. The primary audience for research also differs with researchers identifying the academic community as their primary audience while policymakers and practitioners see the audience as wider to include politicians, civil servants and other practitioners.

Some commentators, such as Feldman, have argued that the difference in perspective between researchers and policymakers has resulted in both acting "like strangers in the night, dimly aware of each other's presence" (1999, p. 48).

Lomas (2000) suggests that relationships can become confrontational, with researchers criticizing the demands of the policymakers while policymakers may dismiss the nuances of research findings. Others such as Bryant (2002) argue that there may be a deliberate agenda driving the distance between research and policy. He cites examples from health policy, where he asserts that no amount of evidence can lead to policy change where the political climate is unwilling to change. Whatever the degree of distance that exists between research, policy and practice communities, it is essential that investment of time and resources in relationship building is recognized as part of the solution. Innvaer et al. (2002) advocate the value of ongoing two-way communication between researchers and policymakers to facilitate the use of research evidence. Lomas (2007) agrees with this position as long as such interactions are of a quality that actually drives research into practice. Others suggest that the research/policy knowledge exchange process can be enhanced through the use of carefully designed software tools (Hammill, Harvey & Echeverria, 2013; Milne et al., 2014).

Knowledge exchange in Irish research, policy and practice

Attention to the personal and the communicative dimensions highlight the fact that knowledge exchange for impact is a social rather than a technical endeavour. It is not about translating research findings into guidelines or checklists – it is about utilizing the research evidence to explore and interrogate existing policy, policy goals and development activity. The iterative nature of consultation based upon research in children's policymaking in Ireland has, perhaps unconsciously, contributed to the development of better knowledge exchange activity in that it allowed for deeper engagement with conceptual ideas emerging from research, illustrating their relevance for both policy and practice (Duignan, 2011). A particular example of this activity was the work of the Centre for Early Childhood Development and Education (CECDE) (2002–2008), which facilitated and delivered both academic research and policy research and development and made particularly effective use of consultative processes which brought together stakeholders engaged in research, policy and practice. This forum for debate and robust exchange of perspectives recognized knowledge exchange as an essential feature for policy development that would lead to meaningful change in practice. Much of the work of the CECDE, in particular that which culminated in the publication of *Síolta, the National Quality Framework for Early Childhood Education* (2006), was premised on the philosophy, grounded in change management theory, that the benefits of engaging in collaborative policymaking is the sense of ownership that it engenders in all those charged with development and implementation strategies (CECDE, 2006; Duignan et al., 2007).

A lasting legacy of the work of the CECDE, regardless of the factors influencing the research/policy and practice divide, was that in the context of addressing the promotion of evidence-informed policy making and practice, researchers must understand that there are actions they can take to facilitate knowledge exchange without compromising the integrity of research. Hall (1993) has described a typology of policy change which provides insight for the research community intent upon effecting knowledge exchange within the arena of policy and practice. The typology identifies three levels of change:

- First order change – normal policy change which is characterized by slight variation, incremental with a continuation of past policies;
- Second order change – gradual paradigmatic policy change through the design of, for instance, new policy tools to meet new but gradual changes;
- Third order change – paradigmatic policy change characterized by fundamental new policy direction underpinned by new ways of thinking.

The argument is made that for paradigmatic change there is a need for cultural change, and this can only come about if researcher and policymakers work together and discuss evidence-based policy development from their various perspectives, each identifying the challenges, barriers and opportunities they foresee in a realistic and respectful way (Wolfe, O'Donoghue-Hynes & Hayes, 2013).

Enhancing direct and indirect impact of research on policymaking and practice

In addition to the CECDE work programme, a range of other research and policymaking activities in Ireland have also demonstrated the potential success for effective knowledge exchange. For instance, inward investment from the European Structural Funds (ESF) has driven the transformation of provision of early childhood education and care (ECEC) services with a view to supporting equity of access for parents to labour force participation in the burgeoning economy. Advocacy for children's rights has gained momentum, albeit within the specific context of historical child abuse scandals. This culminated in 2015 with the amendment of the Constitution (Ireland, 1937) to incorporate an explicit acknowledgement of children as individual rights holders. In all of these instances effective knowledge exchange between research and policymaking was supported by extensive iterative consultation processes, which characterized both research and policymaking activity in relation to the development of particular national children's policy at this time, for example, occupational role profiles for the early childhood workforce (DJELR, 2002), *Síolta, the National Quality Framework for Early Childhood Education* (CECDE, 2006; DES, 2010) and *Aistear, the Early Childhood Curriculum Framework* (National Council for Curriculum and Assessment (NCCA), 2009).

The objective of consultation was to afford diverse stakeholders in national policy and practice the opportunity to have influence on the final policy decision and in doing so to promote greater cohesion in the delivery of practice arising from policy change. The role of research in these processes was clearly defined for each stage of the policymaking process, and usually took the following pattern: step 1 – review of pertinent research literature to establish the evidence-based rationale for the policy; step 2 – completion of a research and development programme which could involve a wide variety of research activity usually including evaluation; step 3 – distillation of the research evidence and formulation of national policy recommendations.

Consultation, characterized by information sharing and debate, was stipulated at all stages of the process. This structure afforded the opportunity for sustained interchange between researchers, practitioners and policymakers. This allowed for the traditional distance between these usually separate domains to be overcome, primarily through the establishment of relationships, which centred on the shared common agenda of improving the situation of children. The DCYA published the *National Strategy for Research and Data on Children's Lives 2011–2016*, which explicitly recognizes the importance of knowledge transfer through its commitment to establish a national database of children's research (2011, p. 12). In the ensuing period to date, consultation has become a regular feature of national policy development and, with the advent of increased state subvention for the provision of services for children, the capacity for engaging in such opportunities has also increased across diverse stakeholder groups. However, vigilance is required on all sides so that the consultation process does not deteriorate into a tokenistic exercise. Internationally, comparisons can be made to the work of organizations such as the Innocenti Centre in Florence, which gathers evidence and knowledge on children world-wide with the aim of sharing information towards improving both social and economic policy for vulnerable children everywhere.

Challenges for knowledge exchange

Collaborative processes afforded by consultation in national policymaking also served to highlight several challenges for knowledge exchange between research, policy and practice. The first of these is the diversity in children's services provision in Ireland. This is a direct outcome of traditional national policymaking based on the principle of subsidiarity, that is, that the State should fund through the auspices of a range of third parties (community, voluntary and private organizations) rather than directly provide a wide range of social services (Fanning, 2004). The lack of coherence across service provision for children and the delivery organizations could be accounted for by the fact that policy underpinning service delivery was made at local or institutional level and was not referenced to any national policy agenda. Government departments, even those with an obvious remit for the provision of public services for children and families – education, health and social protection – did not have a tradition of interdepartmental cooperation towards policy development, and it was not unusual for one department to have limited involvement in policy development activity initiated by another even where the public services arising might be targeted at the same population group. Some effort has been made to overcome this challenge, in particular through the co-location of one business unit attached to one government department in the premises of another – for example, Early Years Education Policy Unit co-located with the DCYA. However, it has been argued that co-location alone will not lead to integrated policy development without careful planning (Hayes, 2010).

Despite some progress in recent times, challenges for knowledge exchange remain in Ireland and elsewhere. These are heightened given that sustaining the fledgling collaborative processes detailed above in an economic and political environment characterized by rationalization and recession has proved unsuccessful, as evidenced in particular by the closure of the CECDE in 2008. In the absence of the forum for exchange across different professional and policy groups provided by the activities of this organization, traditional barriers to collaboration across research, policy and practice arenas have become apparent. In addition to historical and current social, political, cultural and economic influences, there continue to be challenges that arise from the separate nature of the professional cultures associated with ECEC stakeholders in the knowledge exchange process.

Tensions between the research community and policymakers regarding the challenge of maintaining scientific rigour in the research process and ensuring timely relevance to policymaking can inhibit the development of open and trusting relationships. Issues relating to who should translate research findings (and maintain the scientific rigour in the interpretation and the main messages), and who should arrange or manage the knowledge brokering/exchange, become problematic if the agenda of all stakeholders is not fully appreciated and respected. Further, the sharing of the knowledge with those stakeholders in the practice domain is compromised by such tensions, and can impact on the receptiveness of the practice context to the knowledge generated through research. Perception of dissonance between research output and policy that governs practice can inhibit any knowledge exchange at the practice level. A recent example of this is the implementation deficit following the publication of *Síolta* and *Aistear* frameworks in the field of early childhood education and care. The absence of clear policy direction regarding the status of these research-based practice frameworks contributed to the creation of a hiatus in their take-up in practice. In the context of such complex sets of variables, each of which has the potential to impact on the success or failure of knowledge exchange across the fields of research, policy and practice, the concept of knowledge brokering becomes increasingly relevant.

Knowledge brokering

The idea of knowledge brokering was pioneered by Johnathan Lomas at the Canadian Health Services Research Foundation as a response to the 'know–do gap' between research policy and practice. It has been defined as "the active process that links researchers and decision makers (or practitioners) so that they are better able to 'understand each other's goals and professional culture, influence each other's work, forge new partnerships, and use research-based evidence'" (Canadian Health Services Research Foundation, 2008, cited in Goldfeld, 2010, p. 3).

Knowledge brokering has a specific remit and recognizes that creating knowledge and formulating policy are two different processes. The focus is to assist the interactions between researcher and policymaker. This approach can include some or all of the following activity: organizing joint forums; building trust; identifying common goals and mutual opportunities; clarifying information needs; synthesizing research information; sharing information; monitoring impact (van Kammen et al., 2006). The potential of this activity is the effective achievement of knowledge exchange towards evidence-informed decision-making. Dobbins et al. (2009) reviewed the role of knowledge brokering in the development of Canadian health policy with a randomized control trial across three research projects. Knowledge brokering activities were classified into the following categories:

> Initial and ongoing needs assessments; scanning the horizon; knowledge management; knowledge translation and exchange, network development,

> maintenance, and facilitation; facilitation of individual capacity development in evidence informed decision making; and facilitation of and support for organizational change.
>
> (p. 1)

In this study, the outcomes for knowledge exchange for evidence-informed decision-making across the three programmes were examined. The researchers found that only one of the three research programmes had knowledge brokering factored in to the programme. The insight afforded by this research highlighted the critical importance of personal relationship building and, as a corollary, the personal communication skills of the knowledge broker in the knowledge brokering process. It also revealed the need to put in place mechanisms (such as networks) to facilitate and sustain knowledge sharing. The researchers also concluded that knowledge brokering takes time if real relationships of trust are to be established.

This final point suggests that the lack of experience of all stakeholders in knowledge exchange processes is a real and tangible barrier that requires targeted investment of time and resources to overcome. This investment would build the capacity in a range of skills in support of effective knowledge exchange across research policy and practice domains. Despite ambitions to get practitioners and policymakers to use research findings as facts to inform their work, Lomas argues that researchers are not organized to influence policy and practice, and policymakers and practitioners are not receptive towards utilizing research findings (Lomas, 2007). In fact, he has found that the health research world favours grant applications and publication over knowledge synthesis and engagement with the health service, and points out that while researcher to researcher communication is common and well organized, researcher to practitioner dialogue remains poorly organized and rare. He does cite some examples of good practice, such as the UK National Institute for Health and Clinical Excellence (NICE) and the knowledge transfer unit of the Scottish Executive Health Department described by Clark and Kelly (2005). More recently, Goldfeld (2010) has argued that for knowledge brokering to be successful the knowledge broker must have the capacity to engage with a variety of opportunities which have potential to influence decision-making processes. She also argues that there is both an art and a science to knowledge brokering and concludes that "we should not underestimate the importance of the art of persuasion and communication in brokering the science of evidence" (2010, p. 1).

Once again, the personal attributes of successful knowledge brokers are highlighted. These have been discussed in the literature and generally include some or all of the following: that they be entrepreneurial, credible, clear communicators; that they understand both cultures (academic and policy); that they be facilitators and assessors of relevant research in a variety of forms; and that they understand the principles of adult learning (Clark and Kelly, 2005; Lomas, 2007; Goldfeld, 2010).

This skill set reflects the challenging and complex role of the knowledge broker and suggests that access to skilled intervention in this area cannot be left to chance and must be planned for and resourced. In a review of knowledge brokers in the health services in Canada, Lomas (2007) found that 30 per cent are based in universities, 10 per cent in foundations or research funding agencies and the remaining 60 per cent within the health services. The job of a knowledge broker as identified by Lomas (2007) includes 30 per cent knowledge transformation (reading and disseminating research), 20 per cent intermediation (linking researchers and decision makers) and the remaining 50 per cent in management and/or teaching duties (reflecting the usually part-time nature of the work).

It is rare that the knowledge brokering role can be clearly identified within either a research or policymaking context as a fully evolved and valued professional activity. In the experience of these authors, more often it is an activity tacked on to the end of a research programme or assigned to a junior staff member in a policymaking team. Some progress in establishing a clear identity for the knowledge exchange/knowledge broker has been made in Scotland. Clark and Kelly (2005) have identified that the role of knowledge brokers is often seen as part of the academic role. However, they comment that "ambiguity and hybridity are features of emerging knowledge exchange roles – the defining feature of these roles is that KE or KB is an essential or core responsibility and takes up a significant proportion of the post holders time" (2005, p. 4). In evaluating the impact of knowledge brokering work in practice, Fisher notes that the:

> challenge for building a broader understanding of the impact of knowledge brokering is to overcome the differences and the context specific nature of a lot of the work and instead identify the synergies and similarities. If we are able to identify synergies in the outcomes that KB work is intended to achieve then we may be able to build up a picture of what kind of KB interventions work better in what contexts.
>
> (2012, p. 3)

In his review of knowledge brokering in health research, Eleuze (2015) argues that studies have shown some success in knowledge brokering, but calls for more research into the potential role of library and information science professionals in this arena.

Knowledge brokering in Ireland

The goal of effective knowledge exchange and brokering in support of evidence-informed policymaking in Ireland is facing particular challenges. Whilst the successes of evidence-informed policymaking of the past decade are still fresh for many researchers and policymakers, the economic collapse of 2008 placed severe restrictions on resources to continue to build upon these. An example of this is the recent closure due to funding cuts of the Irish Nonprofits Knowledge Exchange (INKEx), which had a remit to provide a comprehensive data repository for the non-profit sector.

What this and similar retrenchment in funding activity means for knowledge exchange is that there is limited opportunity to consolidate the learning on effective knowledge exchange into a set of actions which would support the establishment of a distinct knowledge brokering agency such as that in Canada, where there is a trusted independent Canadian Health Services Research Foundation, or the Scottish model, where researchers and knowledge brokers are embedded within the Scottish Executive Department of Health (Clark & Kelly, 2005). However, despite the difficult economic situation in Ireland, there are still possible routes to ensuring that knowledge brokering and the necessary capacity building in this regard across all stakeholders can be managed. A range of organizations have potential in this regard.

The Centre for Effective Services (CES)

This organization was established in 2008 with joint funding from two government departments and the Atlantic Philanthropies. To date, their work programme has focused on the following:

- Policy Advice and Implementation Support
- Programme Design, Implementation and Practice Development
- Evaluation, Quality and Outcomes
- Knowledge and Communications

Their expressed mission is to "work with others to connect and support the implementation of effective policy, efficient systems and good practice, using the best available evidence, so that children, young people, families and communities thrive" (CES, 2012, p. 4). This clearly is in line with a knowledge exchange/knowledge brokering agenda, and as they described in their *CES Strategy 2012–2014*:

> One way of describing CES is as a think and do tank. We make relevant, usable evidence available to policy makers, service commissioners and providers. We help them to generate evidence through their own practices and work with them to support the implementation of effective policy, efficient systems and good practice. CES does not promote particular services, programmes or organisations. Our agenda is to achieve the best possible outcomes for children, young people, families and communities.
>
> (2012, p. 5)

The CES website elaborates in specific detail their Knowledge Exchange and Communications function, with the following goals being identified:

- Monitor: To monitor key research findings, government publications and policies, media coverage concerning children, young people, families and community (CYPFC) issues;
- Inform: To inform the work of CES staff and external stakeholders on latest information to improve services for CYPFC and influence policy and practice reform in areas impacting on CYPFC;
- Knowledge Exchange: To increase the likelihood that research evidence will be used in policy and practice decisions and to exchange latest information with stakeholders to use in making evidence-informed decisions;
- Persuade: To reinforce or change our stakeholders' interpretation about a particular topic based on evidence;
- Network: To build relationships through identifying a network of CES stakeholders in a range of external organisations;
- Support: To support our stakeholders on an ongoing basis and to build their own knowledge and communications systems.

(www.effectiveservices.org)

The CES state that they will aim to deliver on these goals through a series of knowledge and communications outputs.

Children's Research Network for Ireland and Northern Ireland

Another potential agent for the development of knowledge exchange/brokering activity in Ireland is the Children's Research Network for Ireland and Northern Ireland. Once again, it is funded by government in partnership with philanthropy, and seeks to support the research community in Ireland and Northern Ireland to better understand and improve the lives of children and young people by creating and maintaining an inclusive, independent, non-profit network through which information, knowledge, experience, learning and skills can be shared. Whilst their focus is more specifically targeted at the research community, the potential for integrating capacity building relating to effective knowledge exchange/brokering is obvious.

The major challenge for the both CES and the Children's Research Network is that their funding is project-based and not mainstream, with government investment being predicated upon being matched by that of the philanthropic foundation. Given that this organization has recently announced a winding down of their funding activity in Ireland, similar difficulties to that of other project based policy initiatives may be faced in sustaining the achievements of the CES in the long term.

Health Service Executive, Health Intelligence Unit

What may have greater potential to sustain capacity building in knowledge exchange/brokering is the work of mainstream agencies, which have both a research and policy development remit. The Health Service Executive, Health

Intelligence Unit is an example of such an agency. Health Intelligence is the development and use of knowledge to support decision-making to improve the health of the population. The Health Intelligence Team works to support the health system in making evidence-informed decisions for better health and social care. The stated objectives of the team are:

- Development of evidence-based analyses, products, reports, surveys and methodologies that inform key strategic and operational decision-making needs, including further use and development of the Health Intelligence Ireland information system which is currently supporting development of NQAIS (the National Quality Assurance Intelligence System);
- Enabling health service staff use a range of health intelligence, evidence and knowledge for health through information and knowledge systems, facilitation of groups and teams in decision-making change processes, interventions to get research into practice and targeted skills training;
- Enabling Research and Development in the health system through direct working with internal HSE research structures and linkages with external research bodies (participation in steering groups and authorship of research papers).

(www.hse.ie/eng/about/Who/clinical/Health_Intelligence/Health_Intelligence_Work/)

Their stated priorities for the future include "working directly in an advisory, facilitation, and project management role with clinical programmes and care group service leads on key pieces of work" (www.hse.ie/eng/about/Who/clinical/Health_Intelligence/Health_Intelligence_Work/). There is a clear match here between this goal and that of knowledge exchange.

Irish Research Council

In a similar vein, there is a stipulation around knowledge exchange in research programmes funded through the Irish Research Council. The Research Council operates research funding initiatives which support talented researchers in their early stage career formation across Master's, Doctoral and Postdoctoral levels. The emphasis of the funding programmes is on exploratory research aimed at yielding new concepts, findings and innovations within Ireland. Knowledge exchange has become a requirement for much research funding through the Irish Research Council, and in 2010 the then Irish Research Council for the Humanities and Social Sciences launched the Knowledge Exchange Activities strand funding various knowledge-exchange initiatives. In addition, the Irish Research Council has been offering research funding in partnership with different government departments under specific policy relevant themes.

Post-recession potential

In more recent years the global economic crisis has prompted the initiation of measures within governments to ensure more efficient and effective use of resources, including knowledge. This has primarily been part of a performance review agenda aiming to make decision-making and allocation of public funds more effective and efficient. In Ireland, this is manifest in the increased attention of policymakers to knowledge management as an essential feature of public sector reform. In strategies developed across various government departments, there is an understanding of the value of "identifying, capturing, sorting, storing, sustaining, applying, sharing and renewing knowledge to improve an organisation's performance" (Al-Khouri, 2014, p. 11). Recognizing the value of both explicit and tacit knowledge, systems and structures are being developed to allow for greater coherence and coordination across public policy development. Such developments, which demonstrate a 'readiness for change' in relation to knowledge management, have the potential to create opportunities for knowledge exchange and knowledge brokering processes to find new relevance (Weiner, 2009). Examples of these opportunities being successfully explored can be identified in international literature. In Scotland, reforms in the National Health Service have drawn upon knowledge services to inform all stages of planning, implementation and evaluation (Morton, 2013). Advances in brokering relationships between research and policy have also been identified in health systems across Europe (Lavis and Catallo, 2014), and in Canada decision-making in relation to health service reform has identified knowledge exchange as a central support for government decision making (Hillmer, 2016).

Conclusion

If the best interests of children and young people are to be represented in national policymaking, it is evident that knowledge exchange and knowledge brokering across the domains of research, policy and practice must be effective. This requires researchers to consider communication beyond those perhaps more readily considered channels, which were considered in Chapter 9. There have been some successes in Ireland over the past two decades which, whether deliberately or unconsciously, incorporated good practice in support of knowledge exchange. Such activities included time and resources dedicated to knowledge brokering through relationship building and iterative consultation, which facilitated deeper engagement with research in the context of policy and practice development. Such developments need further nurturing towards mutual understanding and respect across research, policy and practice professionals, and should be built on to support initiatives strengthening knowledge exchange and knowledge brokering as core professional activities across these domains. Whilst there are some agencies articulating a specific brief in this regard, during periods of recession they are particularly vulnerable. In this context the primary objective must be to ensure that the mainstream adopts effective knowledge exchange as a core activity and strives to build capacity in this regard. As the research literature on knowledge exchange demonstrates, the benefits of capacity building will accrue to all.

References

Al-Khouri, A.M. (2014) 'Fusing knowledge management into the public sector: A review of the field and case of the Emirates Identity Authority', *Information and Knowledge Management*, 4(4), pp. 23–74.

Bryant, T. (2002) 'Role of knowledge in public health and health promotion policy change', *Health Promotion International*, 17(1), pp. 89–98.

Canadian Health Services Research Foundation (CHSRF) (2008) *Glossary of knowledge exchange terms as used by the foundation.* Canadian Health Services Research Foundation: Ottawa. Available from www.chsrf.ca/keys/glossary_e.php>.

Canadian Health Services Research Foundation (CHSRF) (2003) *The theory and practice of knowledge brokering in Canada's health system.* Canadian Health Services Research Foundation: Ottawa. Available from www.chsrf.ca/brokering/pdf/Theory_and_Practice_e.pdf.

Centre for Early Childhood Development and Education (CECDE) (2006) *Síolta, the national quality framework for early childhood education in Ireland.* Dublin: CECDE.

Centre for Effective Services (CES) (2012) *CES strategy, better evidence, better outcomes, 2012–2014.* Dublin: CES.

Clark, G. & Kelly, L. (2005) *New directions for knowledge transfer and knowledge brokerage in Scotland: Office of Chief Researcher Knowledge Transfer Team briefing paper.* Edinburgh: Scottish Executive Social Research.

Datta, A. (2012) 'Deliberation, dialogue and debate: Why researchers need to engage with others to address complex issues', *Institute of Development Studies Special Issue: New Roles in Communication in Development?*, 43(5), pp. 9–16.

Department of Children and Youth Affairs (DCYA) (November,2013). 'Minister Fitzgerald updates Dáil on pre-school quality improvements'. Dublin: DCYA. Available from www.dcya.gov.ie/viewdoc.asp?Docid=3019&CatID=11&mn=&StartDate=01+January+2013.

Department of Children and Youth Affairs (DCYA) (2011) *The national strategy for research and data on children's lives 2011–2016.* Dublin: Government Publication Office.

Department of Education and Skills (DES) (2010) *Síolta: The national quality framework for early childhood education.* 2nd edn. Dublin: Government Publications Office.

Department of Justice, Equality and Law Reform (DJELR) (2002) *Model framework for education, training and professional development in the early childhood care and education sector.* Dublin: Government Stationery Office.

Dobbins, M. *et al.* (2009) 'A description of a knowledge broker role implemented as part of a randomized controlled trial evaluating three knowledge translation strategies', *Implementation Science*, 2009(4), p. 23. doi:10.1186/1748-5908-4-23

Duignan, M. (2011) *The growth of professionalism in early childhood care and education in Ireland.* Doctoral Thesis, University College Cork.

Duignan, M. *et al.* (2007) *Síolta: The national quality framework for early childhood education.* Paper presented at the CECDE International Conference, Dublin. Available from www.cecde.ie/english/pdf/conference_papers/Siolta_VIP.pdf.

Eleuze, N. (2015) 'Evaluating the effectiveness of knowledge brokering in health research: A systematised review with some bibliometric information', *Health Information Library Journal*, 32(3), pp. 168–181. doi:10.1111/hir.12097

Fanning, B. (2004) 'Communitarianism, social capital and subsidiarity', in Fanning, B. *et al.* (eds), *Theorising Irish social policy.* Dublin: University College Dublin Press, pp. 42–61.

Feldman, S. (1999) 'Perspective: Strangers in the night: Research and managed mental health care', *Health Affairs,* 18(5), pp. 48–51.

Fisher, C. (2012) *Evaluating the impact of knowledge brokering work: Analysis of an e-discussion on the knowledge brokers' forum.* Brighton: Institute of Development Studies.

Goldfeld, S. (2010) 'The art and science of influence: Reflections from the boundary', in Bammer, G., Michaux, A. & Sanson, A. (eds) *Bridging the 'know–do' gap. Knowledge brokering to improve child wellbeing.* Canberra: ANU E Press. The Australian National University. Available from http://epress.anu.edu.au?p=681.

Hall, P.A. (1993) 'Policy paradigms, social learning, and the state: The case of economic policymaking in Britain', *Comparative Politics,* 25(3), pp. 275–296.

Hammill, A., Harvey, B. & Echeverria, D. (2013) 'Paper. Knowledge for action: an analysis of the use of online climate knowledge brokering platforms', *Knowledge Management for Development Journal*, 9(1), pp. 72–92.

Hayes, N. (2010) 'Childcare? Early childhood education and care? Towards an integrated early years policy for young children in Ireland', *Early Years: An International Journal of Research and Development*, 30(1), pp. 67–78.

Hayes, N. (2006) 'A decade of reflection: Early childhood care and education in Ireland 1996–2006', in Hayes, N. & Bradley, S. (eds) *A decade of reflection: Early childhood care and education in Ireland 1996–2006.* Proceedings of Centre for Social and Educational Research Early Childhood Care and Education Seminar Series 1, November, 2006, pp. 3–10. Available from www.cser.ie.

Hillmer, M. (2016) Health services research and policy making in Ontario. Presentation to the Canadian Knowledge Transfer and Exchange Community of Practice Toronto Chapter. January 2016. http://ktecop.ca/wordpress/wp-content/uploads/KTECOP-Health-Services-Research-20160119.pdf.

Innvaer, S. *et al.* (2002) 'Health policy-makers' perceptions of their use of evidence: A systematic review', *Journal of Health Service Research Policy,* 7, pp. 239–244.

Ireland (1937) *Bunreacht na hÉireann = Constitution of Ireland.* Dublin: Oifig an tSoláthair/Stationary Office.

Lavis, J.N. & Catallo, C. (eds) (2014) *Bridging the worlds of research and policy in European health systems.* Copenhagen, Denmark: WHO Regional Office for Europe.

Lomas, J. (2007) 'The in-between world of knowledge brokering', *British Medical Journal*, 334(7585), pp. 129–132.

Lomas, J. (2000) 'Using "linkage and exchange" to move research into policy at a Canadian Foundation', *Health Affairs,* 19, pp. 236–240.

Lyall, C. (2008) *A short guide to designing interdisciplinary research and practice. Briefing note 6.* Edinburgh: Institute for the Study of Sciences technology and Innovation.

Milne, B.J., *et al.* (2014) 'A collaborative approach to bridging the research-policy gap through the development of policy advice software', *Evidence and Policy*, 10(1), pp. 127–136.

Morton, S. (2013) Evidencing the impact of knowledge services in the NHS in Scotland. Presentation to the Ontario Institute for Studies in Education. September 2013. www.ktecop.ca/resource-library/presentations/evidencing-the-impact-of-knowledge-services-in-the-nhs-in-scotland/

Moser, H. & Zebra, V. (2011) 'Learning community – Immigrants as educational facilitators pave the way for immigrants to access lifelong learning', European Commission Grant Ref. 504 367–2009-LLP-DE-GRUNDTVIG-GMP. Berlin: BGZ. http://bgz-berlin.de/en/projects-and-products/project-overview/learning-community.html

National Council for Curriculum and Assessment (NCCA) (2009) *Aistear, the early childhood curriculum framework*. Dublin: NCCA.

Richardson, V. (1999) 'Children and social policy', in Quin, S. *et al.* (eds) *Contemporary Irish social policy*. Dublin: University College Dublin Press, pp. 170–199.

van Kammen, J., de Savigny, D. & Sewankambo, N. (2006) 'Using knowledge brokering to promote evidence-based policy-making: The need for support structures', *Bulletin of WHO*, August 2006, 84(8), pp. 608–612.

Weiner, B.J. (2009) 'A theory of organisational readiness for change', *Implementation Science*, 4, p. 67.

Wolfe, T., O'Donoghue-Hynes, B. & Hayes, N. (2013) 'Rapid change without transformation: The dominance of a national policy paradigm over international influences on ECEC development in Ireland 1995–2012', *International Journal of Early Childhood*, 45(2), pp. 191–205.

11 Overcoming the ethical and practical challenges associated with archiving qualitative and quantitative data

Tara Murphy, Aileen O'Carroll, Suzanne Guerin and Jane Gray

Introduction

There has been a significantly increased interest in and practice relating to data archiving in recent years. Doorn and Tjalsma (2007) suggest that the increasing role of computers in research has been a key influence in this growth. Similarly, the National Academy of Sciences (2009) proposes that the rapid growth of digital technology and communication has prompted an exponential increase in the volume of data produced by researchers. This has resulted in the need for more refined data management procedures and systems to ensure their integrity and proper stewardship (National Academy of Sciences, 2009). From a research commissioner's perspective, there is an increased emphasis on reporting research that is credible, robust, transparent and accessible (Greenbaum, 2009; Kretser, Murphy & Dwyer, 2017; Lupia & Elman, 2014). For example, Kretser, Murphy and Dwyer (2017) noted the significant efforts of organizations in the United States, including the National Institutes of Health (NIH) and the National Academy of Sciences, to improve the scientific integrity of research through various methods, including data sharing. Moving closer to home, funders such as the UK's Economic and Social Research Council (ESRC), Wellcome Trust and Cancer Research UK promote the accessibility of data to maximize public benefit while preserving intellectual property, confidentiality and data protection (The Digital Curation Centre, accessed 14/02/17). Therefore, researchers must be in a position to consider the ethical and practical issues involved in the process of data archiving.

At the same time, there have been significant historical and social changes in the depth and breadth of the ethical issues researchers must consider, both generally and in relation to archiving. A paper published by the Hastings Centre (Albala, Doyle & Appelbaum, 2010) reviewed the information submitted by applicants to one Institutional Review Board over a 25-year period. They noted a decrease in the number of studies where participants were misinformed as to the level of risk involved in the study, and an increase in the length and level of detail contained within the participant information. Corti, Day and Backhouse (2000) also highlight the changing view of covert research since the 1960s and 1970s. While more general ethical issues evident in the research process have been considered in Chapter 3 and Chapter 7 of this text, the intricacies of archiving data for reuse mean that the specific ethical issues in this area warrant consideration. A particular area of change with implications for data archiving is that of data protection, which in Ireland has been driven by the Data Protection Act 1988 and the Data Protection (Amendment) Act 2003 at a national level, as well as the EU Data Protection Directive 95/46/EC. In the UK the Data Protection Act (Office of Public Sector Information, 1998) has had a similar influence. We will discuss the specific issues of data protection in relation to archiving later in this chapter. The key point for now is the potential for this legislation to influence practice in archiving.

With the growth of interest in and practice relating to data archiving in social and economic research, researchers must be in a position to consider the ethical and practical issues involved in the archiving process. Equally, research commissioners should consider data archiving as a pragmatic solution for ensuring the integrity, accessibility and stewardship of the research they fund in accordance with 'open science' principles. This chapter discusses some of those challenges, both generally and with specific emphasis on archiving varieties of research data arising from community change initiatives (CCIs), also referred to as comprehensive community initiatives in some instances. It highlights some of the key concerns raised by researchers about archiving quantitative and qualitative data, most notably informed consent, data ownership and the management of confidentiality and anonymity. Findings are based on a case study of a community initiative to provide instances of where community evaluation research might present some additional challenges relating to archiving, and to identify ways of overcoming those challenges. The chapter concludes with key learning for community organizations, research commissioners, practitioners and researchers that may be considering archiving data for future use.

Benefits of archiving

Before we look at the ethical issues involved in the practice of data archiving, there is a need to recognize some of the ethical debates about the principle of archiving data. Planning to share data has been argued to enhance scientific rigour, and confidence in research findings more generally, in a number of ways. Albright and Lyle (2010) provide an overview of some of the reasons for archiving, including the ability to validate and refine or refute published findings using publically available data, not just to counteract incidents of data falsification, but also in response to the many errors that can occur in the process of analysis. Archiving may ensure greater transparency of data (Carusi & Jirotka, 2009; National Academy of Sciences, 2009) as well as improving methods of data collection and measurement. Sharing data also encourages the development of different approaches and perspectives, facilitating new analyses and interpretations that may not have been anticipated in the original research project.

Data sharing provides additional benefits to data commissioners and research participants. It can reduce costs by avoiding duplication, thereby also reducing the burden on participants associated with multiple data collection efforts. For example, Carusi and Jirotka (2009) highlight the pragmatic reasons for archiving data, including "avoiding the repetition of expensive research by allowing research that has already been carried out to be exploited as fully as possible" (p. 286). Similarly, Greene-Moton et al. (2006) highlight the negative impact of 'parachuting' researchers into communities already overburdened with multiple research projects, which can increase feelings of mistrust and disillusion among community members.

While Corti, Day and Backhouse (2000) mention the perception that archiving is in the public interest, there is a debate that contrasts with the ethical principle that archiving reduces the burden on participants from unnecessary repeat data collection. This contrasting argument suggests that use of archived data represents a potential breach of privacy and the aforementioned data protection legislation. Grinyer (2009) discusses the perception that archiving qualitative data, in particular, runs contrary to expectations that secondary analysis requires additional consent. She goes on to conclude that participants' expectations, and specifically how individuals may want their data to be used, are key principles. Rahu and McKee (2008) discuss the specific issue of privacy in relation to analysis of epidemiological data in Estonia, where the EU Data Protection Directive resulted in an outcry by public health researchers regarding its implications for the analysis of existing datasets. Interestingly, the Irish Office of the Data Protection Commissioner advises that "any use or disclosure must be necessary for the purpose(s) or compatible with the purpose(s) for which you collect and keep the data. You should ask yourself whether the data subject would be surprised to learn that a particular use of or disclosure of their data is taking place" (n.d., p. 8). This might suggest that data collected for research could be re-used for further research (as these are compatible uses), but again the expectations of participants are central to the judgement, reflecting the collaborative and responsive approach to community research considered in Chapter 2 but also evident throughout this text.

The important implication, then, is that researchers have a social and custodial duty to the participants who contributed data in the course of a project. The debate, however, seems to move between seeing archiving and sharing as assisting researchers in discharging that obligation and seeing it as a failure to protect the rights of those same participants. Despite this debate, the benefits of sharing are now generally accepted in relation to quantitative data, and the practice of archiving such data is relatively uncontroversial amongst social scientists. However, there are some challenges and concerns regarding archiving that apply to both quantitative and qualitative data, and it is to these challenges that this chapter now turns.

Key challenges to archiving

The existing literature highlights the debates regarding the different challenges associated with archiving qualitative and quantitative data, with some researchers arguing that quantitative data are more easily and more appropriately archived (Parry & Mauthner, 2004). Nevertheless, the issue of ethics arises in relation to both types of data. The OECD's *Declaration on Access to Research Data from Public Funding* (2004) highlights recognition of ethical issues as a key principle in developing access to archived data. Interestingly, a survey of Canadian researchers' attitudes to archiving highlighted ethical issues as a key concern (Perry, 2008). Similar concerns in relation to qualitative data are addressed in the discussion by Corti, Day and Backhouse (2000).

Albright and Lyle (2010) comment on the issue of privacy in relation to archiving, highlighting concerns regarding the impact of modern computing technology on the potential to identify participants in quantitative research using advanced data analysis algorithms. They describe how these concerns have led to masking potentially identifiable data in order to ensure that individual records cannot be identified. They cite a number of commonly used techniques such as data swapping, microaggregation and adding random observations that have been used to protect privacy in archived data. Clearly these techniques do not transfer easily to qualitative data. However, there has been a significant amount of discussion on the idea of privacy and anonymity when archiving qualitative data.

Parry and Mauthner (2004) highlight some of the challenges in anonymizing qualitative data, given the frequency with which detailed field notes are included as part of the analysed data, and also as a result of the frequent use of smaller, more identifiable samples in qualitative research. Interestingly, they comment that the removal of data to protect participants' identities or the archiving of incomplete datasets can actually undermine the usefulness of the data by compromising its validity. A further intricacy in this debate that is unique to qualitative research is the issue of researcher anonymity. Parry and Mauthner (2004) go on to cite the dynamic nature of qualitative research and the likelihood that researchers provide personal information to build rapport as potential influences here. Despite these challenges, Corti, Day and Backhouse (2000) draw on the experience in Qualidata – the Economic and Social Research Council's Qualitative Data Archival Resource Centre – to highlight a range of steps that can be applied to address some of these issues, including the use of restricted access to data, procedures for recontacting participants and guidelines for anonymization of qualitative data (see also Corti et al., 2014).

In addition to privacy and anonymity, another issue central to ethical debates regarding archiving relates to participant consent. Linking this back to the general issue of data protection, it is interesting to note variations in data protection legislation regarding sourcing consent to use data. Parry and Mauthner (2004) report that in the UK the use of data for research purposes falls under an exemption that allows its use without explicit consent (albeit with caveats relating to the potential for 'harm' and the sensitive nature of the data). By contrast, in Ireland one of the key elements of the legislation is that data can be used as long as the use is not at odds with the initial reason for collection, which is often taken as supporting the use of research data for further research. From a general point of view, there can be no doubt that archiving on the basis of informed consent is best practice in this area, and in Ireland researchers are becoming more au fait with the benefits of securing consent to archive data at the outset of studies. However, it is important to consider whether consent to archive truly represents informed consent, as researchers cannot specify the exact way in which a participant's data might be used (Carusi & Jirotka, 2009). Interestingly, Parry and Mauthner (2004) highlight this as particularly problematic with qualitative data, given the developmental and reflexive nature of qualitative research. Corti, Day and Backhouse (2000) stress the importance of clarifying the terms and conditions of future use as much as possible when qualitative data are being archived.

Across the international social science community, many researchers continue to have concerns about archiving, particularly qualitative data (Mauthner & Parry, 2009, see the discussion in Kuula, 2010/2011) and there is now considerable scholarly literature on the debate, which centres on two main areas of concern: (1) whether the re-use of qualitative data is in keeping with some of the fundamental principles of qualitative research; and (2) ethical and legal issues (Heaton, 2008, see also Bishop, 2009). Within this context, the chapter now moves to describe and draw on a specific Irish case study that explored the issue of archiving data from a comprehensive CCI involving children and families across a range of community settings. As we will show, archiving data arising from CCIs may present unique ethical and practical challenges for researchers and research commissioners compared with other types of research projects. The researchers and research commissioners who were consulted as part of the Irish case study articulated many of the same concerns about archiving and sharing qualitative data that have been identified in the literature. However, many also suggested both that the problems were more pronounced in CCIs and that there were additional problems associated with archiving data from such projects.

CCIs were developed as a bottom-up way of responding to the multiple needs of disadvantaged communities in the United States in a coordinated, integrated and collaborative way (Kubisch, 2005). They were established in recognition of the strength of the community to influence the development and well-being of children, young people and their families (Chaskin, 2006), acknowledging the community's capacity to initiate positive community change through the eradication of, for example, social inequality, extreme poverty, poor environmental conditions and the decline of inner-city neighbourhoods, as well as through the delivery of more effective services (Kubisch et al., 2002; Stagner & Duran, 1997). CCIs may be characterized by collaborative partnerships between the community, public and/or private sectors (Kubisch, 2005; Kubisch et al., 2002). CCIs address a range of needs at multiple levels (that is, individual, familial and community) through the implementation of innovative child-, family- and community-focused programmes and initiatives, designed to bring about positive changes in the lives of those living and working in the community (Stagner & Duran, 1997).

Tallaght West Childhood Development Initiative: Case study

The Tallaght West Childhood Development Initiative (CDI) was established as a CCI in 2003 to implement a ten-year programme of activities with local voluntary, statutory and community agencies. CDI is one of three Prevention and Early Intervention Programme (PEIP) sites co-funded by the Atlantic Philanthropies and the Department of Children and Youth Affairs (DCYA) (formerly the Office of the Minister for Children & Youth Affairs). It was never intended to be a long-term project, but rather an organization mandated by its strategy to improve outcomes for children and families. Within this context, one of the key issues for CDI upon its cessation is the secure storage or destruction of research data and documentation arising from its work. During the last number of years, a significant amount of information, including quantitative and qualitative research data, was generated through seven robust evaluations and an epidemiological study, as well as through activities associated with its services. This has required considerable thinking and action around the development of an information management system to oversee the appropriate archiving of data and documentation associated with the CDI. As a result, McGrath and Hanin (2013) developed guidelines and procedures for CDI's data archiving process in line with nationally and internationally agreed best practice for both qualitative and quantitative data.

CDI is strongly committed to the dissemination, application and utilization of research evidence to inform policy and practice. It also positions itself as being an open and transparent organization, accountable to both its funders and the community. Archiving data was identified as one possible strategy for ensuring a greater level of transparency while maximizing the dissemination of learning to other researchers, research commissioners and practitioners. It therefore seemed appropriate for CDI to consider the possibilities for archiving material for future use.

While a number of large-scale studies such as Growing Up in Ireland, the National Longitudinal Study of Children (Trinity College Dublin and the Economic and Social Research Institute), the Millennium Cohort Study (Centre for Longitudinal Studies (UK)) and the Northern Ireland Longitudinal Study (Northern Ireland Statistics and Research Agency) had archived or were beginning the process of archiving research data, there was no known evidence of similar community development organizations in Ireland having formally archived documentation for future use. In light of this, CDI met with two key data archiving institutions, namely the Irish Social Sciences Data Archive (ISSDA) and the Irish Qualitative Data Archive (IQDA), to discuss the feasibility of archiving primarily research and evaluation data with their institutions. The discussion with the ISSDA focused on the way in which quantitative data might be usefully coded and stored until it was suitable for transferring to the archive. The development of a common coding system was suggested as an interface between different project databases. A common coding system had been previously discussed as a way of tracking the progress and impact of the evaluations on children and families. However, an exploration of the potential for developing a coding system identified several logistical difficulties which resulted in this not being pursued.

During this time, a parallel discussion between CDI and the evaluation teams regarding the ownership of evaluation data led to the realization that a discrepancy existed between what the evaluations had been ethically approved for and what the details of their contracts with CDI stated. More specifically, it was automatically understood that intellectual property rights were held by the various evaluation teams. However, one of the stipulations of CDI's funders is that any intellectual property developed, acquired, made or discovered during the course of the evaluation in connection to CDI's programme of activities is solely owned by CDI. The evaluations, as they stood, were unintentionally in breach of their contractual obligations with CDI. As a result, all evaluation teams were asked to resolve this with their ethics committees.

An exploration of the feasibility of archiving evaluation research data arising from community-based initiatives led to a study around archiving and utilization of CDI's qualitative data. This was an innovative and collaborative study between CDI and IQDA, co-funded by CDI and the Irish Research Council for the Humanities and Social Sciences. The study, referred to as RACcER (Re-use and Archiving of Complex Community-based Evaluation Research), resulted in the establishment and dissemination of best practice guidelines for the archiving and re-use of qualitative data (see www.iqda.ie for further details). It coincided with a shared interest in the significance and potential role of qualitative social science data in policy development and evaluation. The purpose of the study was to identify and propose solutions to the challenges associated with archiving complex qualitative data and making it available for re-use, in accordance with international best practice and national research policy objectives. The study took place across three phases: (1) consultation with stakeholders in the wider social science community regarding their experiences, concerns and suggestions in relation to archiving qualitative data; (2) design and implementation of a strategy for archiving internal process data from the CDI evaluations in a manner that took account of stakeholder concerns, while also maximizing the value and potential of the data for re-use by future researchers and service providers; (3) development of a set of recommendations to assist researchers in building the planning and implementation of data archiving into complex qualitative research designs. The potential for archiving qualitative data from CDI's evaluations was explored through individual interviews with members of the evaluation teams in terms of challenges and value. However, several concerns were raised by this group of researchers, echoing those identified in the literature and particularly relating to anonymity, confidentiality and social desirability.

It was therefore agreed that primary qualitative data and any identifiable information (for example, raw interview transcripts, contact details for participants) would not be passed on to CDI but rather stored by the evaluation teams in line with their data protection guidelines. Alternative data sources were identified for archiving, including meeting minutes, structured reports and visual media. Though this type of material is considered different in nature to, for example, interview transcripts, all documents were treated in the same way as raw transcripts. The following section provides a summary of some of the key findings arising from the RACcER project with supporting quotes.

Thirty social science researchers from leading academic institutions in Ireland and Northern Ireland were interviewed as part of the RACcER project in relation to implementation challenges and solutions associated with archiving data (RACcER, 2010). While the focus of the interviews was primarily on archiving qualitative data, many of the issues and solutions identified by the researchers were also applicable to quantitative data. Some of these findings are presented here under broad themes, which have been adapted from Heaton (2008).

Establishing the added value in re-using archived data

Social science researchers have identified several areas where qualitative data sharing and re-use may present different challenges from those presented by quantitative data. For example, there may be a problem of data fit. The objective nature of quantitative research means that its data may be more easily subjected to further statistical analysis. Qualitative research generally entails flexible research designs and unstructured or semi-structured forms of data collection. This raises questions about the extent to which the datasets generated through such methods can be used to answer new or different research questions. The respondents to the RACcER project did articulate concerns about the re-use potential of data from the CDI evaluations, but for reasons less to do with the nature of qualitative data and more to do with the purpose for which the data had been collected and with their function and position as evaluators within the project. Some respondents suggested that if they were diligent in their work, then there was little potential to derive 'added value' from the data: "I'm certainly very diligent about wringing every millilitre of analytical juice out of those datasets".

One respondent indicated that there was often a certain "laziness" about some commissioned research, whereby both commissioners and researchers adopted a minimalist approach that failed to make full use of all the material collected. In this case there might be scope for re-using, but there was a concern that archiving would amount to an admission that the primary researchers had failed to analyse the dataset sufficiently. However, another respondent acknowledged that data could be under-used because "another contract comes on board".

There were divergent views about the re-use potential of evaluation data. Some applied policy researchers expressed the view that, because evaluations tend to be so specific and detailed in relation to a particular project or service, it might be difficult to gain value from the research material in ways that would be applicable to other circumstances. However, other respondents believed that, although very specific data are collected in evaluation research, university-based evaluation teams would also try to include wider research questions associated with the work, and many would have PhD students attached to projects.

The problem of data fit arose in a different way amongst respondents who saw considerable potential value to be gained from exploring the data across the three PEIP sites. A researcher who is familiar with one of the other sites suggested that the data across the three sites were not being collected in such a way that would facilitate cross-site analysis, and believed it unfortunate that there was a general lack of coordination between the research teams working on the different projects.

The importance of context

Many researchers emphasize the importance of context for interpreting and analysing qualitative data, and the difficulties entailed in providing sufficient information on context to enable re-use of archived data. In the context of quantitative data this issue is often addressed with the use of detailed data manuals developed for specific datasets. In addition, it could be argued that the use of standardized measures in quantitative research make re-use easier.

This problem was also mentioned by respondents to the RACcER project. There were concerns that the degree of anonymization required to protect informants within a community-based project would make the archived data "completely useless" to potential re-users. For example, in the CDI context, the job roles held by some individuals would make them fully identifiable. However, the removal of that information would make it difficult, if not impossible, to interpret the transcript of their interview, given that information about the job role would determine the point of view the person was coming from and their relationship with other people they mentioned: "[So] then you do all this anonymization activity, you invest time and money in it, and what you come out with is nothing. If you remove all the contextual information and so on. Then you've got a set of data which would essentially be akin to what was in a report".

The problem of verification

This is, in many ways, the issue that generates most heat in debates about qualitative data archiving, and is one that acquires particular salience in the context of commissioned evaluation research. As Heaton (2008, p. 40) observes:

> Methods of verification derived from positivist-based approaches, which underpin the data sharing imperative in quantitative research, are anathema to many qualitative researchers, for whom alternative methods have been developed to help establish the 'trustworthiness' and authenticity of their work.

In addition to these philosophical concerns, researchers engaged in commissioned work may be more than usually anxious about the potential for damage to their reputations, and to those of the institutions, services and communities involved, following on from secondary analysis of their data.

Some of the respondents emphasized the intrinsically 'political' nature of evaluation research, that of its nature entails judgements of the success or otherwise of initiatives, services or individuals:

> Not only do you have to bring innovative research skills but you are involved from day one in a political exercise ... in a complex set of negotiations with the participants, community groups [...] it also involves the varying sets of expectations that people in the community will have of you ... people's expectations and notions may change over time. You can be involved in a constant process of re-negotiating what's reasonable and what rights various parties have.

Evaluators see their role as involving judgement calls, weighing up the varying points of view and assessing services on that basis. It is a difficult balancing act and there is often a fine line to tread in how reports are written:

> Let's say you do an evaluation and everything is fine with the programme, they have a really good board, people are participating and let's say you have a team that is absolutely dysfunctional ... [From] an evaluation point of view it's hard enough to deal with that kind of stuff but how do you deal with that in an archiving situation, making stuff like that available, like you can't.

For many of our respondents, the potential for using archived data to 'verify' findings in such a 'political' context was either problematic or unacceptable. On the other hand, some interviewees suggested that the archived material could be useful to check back on the research team's work, to determine whether they had been fair and balanced in their interpretations or epistemological standpoints. In this vein, some respondents indicated that they would only be interested in undertaking re-analysis of a dataset if they were particularly unhappy or aggrieved at the outcome of the original analysis. Others suggested that archived material could be used in a way that would apply inter-rater checks to the report. Finally, some respondents were frank about their fears that archiving data would expose them to critique: "To let that go, to other researchers to re-analyse things, maybe they come out with a different paper so there's, kind of like, are you ready for that?"

It should be noted, however, that the counterview was argued very strongly by others. Those who dismissed this risk felt that all researchers should be open to having their work examined and scrutinized by others, and that researchers operating with integrity should be able to defend their analysis, or alternatively admit mistakes where these had occurred. Some felt very strongly that this type of debate over research findings was central to the academic endeavour and contributed to the standing of research, and that researchers should welcome the opportunity to engage with detractors.

Maintaining confidentiality

All researchers planning to make their data available for sharing and re-use must address the issue of how to ensure that any commitments they have made to assure confidentiality to informants are honoured. There are now well-tried and established approaches to addressing this issue within the data archiving community.

However, respondents articulated the view that there were additional risks associated with maintaining confidentiality within an evaluation project centred on a small geographical area "where everybody knows everybody else". Many believed that the removal or substitution of names, places and characteristics would be insufficient to make interviewees unrecognizable. In these environments, the turns of phrase that people use, and the issues or bugbears that they are associated with, would clearly mark them out if a full transcript were archived. Also, people can often be very revealing in interviews, giving a huge level of detail about their lives that would make them easily identifiable.

Respondents also believed that they had a greater than normal level of obligation to preserve the confidentiality of the information provided by their informants, given that the work was being carried out with a marginalized population. There was a strong sense of a duty of care to those whose contribution to research work would potentially be archived. There was a belief among respondents that those coming fresh to research material would not have the same direct relationship with those who had originally participated in the research, and would have less of an obligation to sympathetically reflect their views.

It was also noted that evaluation research may entail an unusually high degree of sensitivity in the information that people are sharing. Some suggested that in this context everything had the potential to be sensitive and that a research team wouldn't necessarily be in a position to make a call about what would or wouldn't be problematic:

> There's [sic] interconnections, there's politics, and there's alliances, and there's, you know, sort of, tensions between people and characters and actors and, [there's] a finite list of characters. I think, in that context, it is challenging about how to anonymize that work and then allow it to be available and maybe you can't, I don't know, maybe that's not possible.

Obtaining informed consent

There were widespread and strong views among respondents that archiving should only be pursued when express consent had been given by participants.

Lack of familiarity with archiving meant that some researchers were dubious about what might be involved in securing such consent: "I don't understand enough about archiving. I wouldn't even be comfortable asking someone to agree to archive the information because I don't know enough about what implications that would have for them".

Most of the RACcER respondents thought that securing retrospective consent for archiving would be impossible, although international evidence – and evidence from the archiving phase of the RACcER project itself – shows that researchers tend to overestimate the difficulties in this regard (Kuula 2010/2011).

Contractual and legal issues (data protection, copyright and data ownership)

Contention around data ownership was a major issue for RACcER respondents, and is likely to be a complicating issue for evaluation projects in general. Due in part to a disagreement between the data commissioners and the evaluation teams in the case of CDI, researchers were particularly sensitive about decision-making processes in relation to archiving, and there was a strong undercurrent of concern that in the event of archiving, research teams would be disenfranchised and overlooked in relation to developing depositor agreements, undertaking anonymization and oversight of data re-use.

Procedures for archiving

In tandem with the consultation with researchers, and as a case study, the RACcER team began the process of identifying and preparing CDI documentation for archiving. The first step was to establish the range and volume of documents potentially available for archiving. There were over 4,000 documents stored electronically by CDI in MS Word, Rich Text Format and PDF format and it was agreed that a smaller sample of material would be selected for archiving. The material was selected on the basis of (a) having low, medium or high sensitivity; (b) having a large but manageable volume; and (c) there being fewer perceived challenges in securing retrospective consent from participants. Minutes from Communities of Practice meetings for three of CDI's services were selected as having low to medium sensitivity and being of a sufficient volume to make the archiving process worthwhile. Communities of Practice are a key support for service providers and include sessions involving invited speakers on relevant topics, case study presentations and facilitated sessions on key issues affecting service delivery. Board minutes were identified as being particularly sensitive and therefore posing specific challenges in terms of anonymization. However, it was agreed that working with these minutes would offer the researchers a valuable opportunity to demonstrate to others the way in which such sensitive documentation could be successfully anonymized and archived. The final set of documents selected for archiving were minutes from CDI management meetings. As with the Board minutes, these were also considered as having medium to high sensitivity. Consent was sought and granted from all but two participants (n=70) to archive the documents (two participants were unreachable). All documents were treated in the strictest confidence by the project team.

In line with international best practice guidelines for archiving qualitative data, an archiving strategy was developed and approved in principle by the CDI Board. The strategy provided the context for archiving, explored potential ethical and security risks associated with various qualitative material and outlined several solutions for managing those risks, including preserving participant privacy and confidentiality. These included restricting access to the data, placing time embargoes on specific anonymized data and implementing license agreements between the depositor (in this case, CDI), the archival unit (IQDA) and the data user. The end-user license agreement was legally binding and ensured that the archived data were used for the sole purposes of the research objectives as outlined by the researcher. A second license agreement was agreed between CDI and the IQDA for transferring, storing and accessing material. This meant that ownership and copyright of the dataset and related contextual material would be transferred to the IQDA in good faith upon the cessation of the CDI.

Finally, over 500 documents were encrypted and transferred to the IQDA using an encryption programme called TruCrypt©. This ensured the safe and secure transfer of electronic material to the archive. Contextual information was also provided to aid with the re-use and interpretation of the data. The reliability of the anonymization process was assessed by both the research team and members of CDI, based on the documents' degree of sensitivity. A key output arising from the RACcER was the development of best practice guidelines in archiving qualitative data (Gray et al., 2011). To conclude, the RACcER project signalled one of the first attempts by an Irish CCI to increase the transparency, accessibility and stewardship of its research in accordance with national and international best practices. Perhaps the most important lesson for the international community is the requirement to build planning to share data into the research management lifecycle from the beginning of any complex community initiative.

Conclusion

The current practice of archiving data from research and evaluation projects is influenced by the various ethical and practical issues associated with the archiving process. This chapter discussed some of the challenges to, and benefits of, archiving both quantitative and qualitative data. For example, archiving data may: validate, refine or refute findings; reduce costs by avoiding duplication; promote the utilization of data for future use, thereby also reducing the burden on participants associated with multiple data collection efforts; and improve methods of data collection and measurement. It may also challenge researchers and data users in terms of ensuring the preservation of participant anonymity and confidentiality.

The chapter drew on findings from a case study of a community initiative to demonstrate instances of where community evaluation research might present some additional challenges relating to archiving, and identified ways of overcoming those challenges. In conclusion, the key learning points include that archiving takes time and requires careful planning and that it has a range of challenges, but equally benefits. Archiving is important that confidentiality and anonymity of participants and organizations are prioritized and maintained at all times and it is also important to agree who has ultimate ownership of the material pre- and post-archiving. Finally, the dissemination and utilization of the archived material is important in terms of maximizing any learning.

Acknowledgements

The RACcER Project was co-funded by the Irish Research Council for the Humanities and Social Sciences and Tallaght West Childhood Development Initiative under the IRCHSS Research Development Initiative, Strand 5, 2008–2009.

References

Albala, I., Doyle, M. & Appelbaum, P.S. (2010) 'The evolution of consent forms for research: A quarter century of changes', *Ethics and Human Research*, 32(3), pp. 7–11.

Albright, J.J. & Lyle, J.A. (2010) 'Data preservation through data archives', *Political Science and Politics*, 43(1), pp. 17–21.

Bishop, L. (2009). 'Ethical sharing and reuse of qualitative data', *Australian Journal of Social Issues*, 44(3), pp. 255–272.

Carusi, A.& Jirotka, M. (2009) 'From data archive to ethical labyrinth', *Qualitative Research*, 9(3), pp. 285–298.

Chaskin, R.J. (2006) 'Family support as community-based practice: Considering a community capacity framework for family support provision', in Dolan, P., Canavan, J. & Pinkerton, J. (eds), *Family support as reflective practice*. London: Jessica Kingsley Publishers, pp. 42–60.

Corti, L., Day, A. & Backhouse, G. (2000) 'Confidentiality and informed consent: Issues for consideration in the preservation of and provision of access to qualitative data archives', *FQS: Forum Qualitative Social Research/Sozialforschung*, 1(3), Article 7. Available from www.qualitative-research.net/index.php/fqs/article/viewArticle/1024/2207.

Corti, L., Van Den Eynden, V. & Bishop, L. (2014). *Managing and sharing research data: A guide to good practice*. London: SAGE.

Doorn, P.& Tjalsma, H. (2007) 'Introduction: Archiving research data', *Archival Science*, 7(1), pp. 1–20.

European Union (1995) *Directive 95/46/EC of the European Parliament and of the Council of 24 October 1995 on the protection of individuals with regard to the processing of personal data and on the free movement of such data*. Available from http://eur-lex.europa.eu/LexUriServ/LexUriServ.do?uri=CELEX:31995L0046:EN:HTML.

Gray, J. *et al.* (2011) 'Best practice in archiving qualitative data.' NIRSA Working Paper Series. No. 65. National University of Ireland Maynooth.

Government of Ireland (1988) *Data Protection Act*. Dublin: The Stationery Office.

Government of Ireland (2003) *Data Protection (Amendment) Act*. Dublin: The Stationery Office.

Greenbaum, D. (2009) 'Research fraud: Methods for dealing with an issue that negatively impacts society's view of science', *Columbia Science and Technology Law Review*, 10, p. 61.

Greene-Moton, E. *et al.* (2006) 'Unit 4: Trust and communication in a CBPR partnership – spreading the "glue" and having it stick', in *The Examining Community-Institutional Partnerships for Prevention Research Group. Developing and sustaining community-based participatory research partnerships: A skill-building curriculum*. Available from www.cbprcurriculum.info.

Grinyer, A. (2009) 'The ethics of the secondary use and further analysis of qualitative data', *Social Research Update*, 56, pp. 1–4.

Heaton, J. (2008) 'Secondary analysis of qualitative data: An overview', *Historical Social Research*, 33(3), pp. 33–45.

Kretser, A., Murphy, D. & Dwyer, J. (2017) 'Scientific integrity resource guide: Efforts by federal agencies, foundations, non-profit organizations, professional societies, and academia in the United States', *Critical Review in Food Science and Nutrition*, 57(1), pp. 163–180

Kubisch, A.C. (2005) 'Comprehensive community building initiatives – ten years later: What we have learned about the principles guiding the work', *New Directions for Youth Development*, 106, pp. 17–26.

Kubisch, A.C. *et al.* (2002) *Voices from the field II: Reflections on comprehensive community change*. Washington, DC: The Aspen Institute.

Kuula, A. (2010/2011) 'Methodological and ethical dilemmas of archiving qualitative data', *IASSIST Quarterly*, 34(3 & 4) and 35(1 & 2), pp. 12–17.

Lupia, A. & Elman, C. (2014) 'Openness in political science: Data access and research transparency: Introduction', *PS: Political Science & Politics*, 47(1), pp. 19–42.

Mauthner, N.S. & Parry, O. (2009) 'Qualitative data preservation and sharing in the social sciences: On whose philosophical terms?' *Australian Journal of Social Issues*, 44(3), pp. 291–307.

McGrath, B. & Hanan, R. (2016) *Sharing social research data in Ireland: A practical toolkit*. Dublin, Ireland: commissioned by Tallaght West Childhood Development Initiative (CDI).

National Academy of Sciences (2009) *Ensuring the integrity, accessibility, and stewardship of research data in the digital age*. Washington, DC: National Academy of Sciences.

OECD (2004) *Final communiqué of the meeting of the OECD committee for scientific and technological policy at ministerial level, 29–30 January 2004,* **Annex 1. Declaration on access to research data from public funding**. Available from www.oecd.org/document/15/0,2340,en_2649_33703_25998799_1_1_1_1,00.htm.

Office of the Data Protection Commissioner (n.d.) *Data Protection Acts 1988 and 2003: A guide for data controllers*. Dublin: Office of the Data Protection Commissioner. Available from www.dataprotection.ie.

Office of Public Sector Information (1998) *Data Protection Act*. London. Available from www.legislation.gov.uk.

Parry, O. & Mauthner, N.M. (2004) 'Whose data are they anyway? Practical, legal and ethical issues in archiving qualitative data', *Sociology*, 38(1), pp. 139–152.

Perry, C.M. (2008) 'Archiving of publicly funded research data: A survey of Canadian researchers', *Government Information Quarterly*, 25, pp. 133–148.

RACcER (2010) *Re-use and archiving of complex community-based evaluation research*. Dublin: Irish Qualitative Data Archive, National University of Ireland Maynooth and Tallaght West Childhood Development Initiative. Further information available from www.iqda.ie/content/raccer-re-use-and-archiving-complex-community-based-evaluation-research.

Rahu, M. & McKee, M. (2008) 'Epidemiological research labelled as a violation of privacy: The case of Estonia', *International Journal of Epidemiology*, 37(3), pp. 678–682.

Stagner, M.W. & Duran, M.A. (1997) 'Comprehensive community initiatives: Principles, practice and lessons learned', *The Future of Children*, 7(2), pp. 132–140.

The Digital Curation Centre. Available from www.dcc.ac.uk/resources/policy-and-legal/overview-funders-data-policies (Accessed on 14 February 2017).

12 Conclusion

Nóirín Hayes and Catherine Comiskey

Introduction

The main aim of this text was to provide the reader with a broad-based guide to the best practice in conducting policy- and practice-relevant research on children, families and communities within a real world context in pragmatic settings. We have embedded the work within theory, the international literature and our own experiences from the Research, Evaluation, Policy and Practice (REPP) Project, which grew out of a joint initiative between The Atlantic Philanthropies (AP) and the Irish government. The REPP project represents a collaboration of individual researchers, practitioners and policymakers actively involved in these areas of research. The detailed outputs from these collaborations and their research projects with children, families and communities can be found throughout the chapters and within the references. Further details can also be found at The Atlantic Philanthropies (www.atlanticphilanthropies.org/subtheme/prevention-early-intervention). This chapter reviews each chapter, draws out the key messages and identifies a number of themes. Taking these themes, the chapter presents four integrating features and brings them together into a model capturing the essential ingredients identified by the book as contributing to best practice for community-based research.

Overview

Across the chapters of this book, development of inter-related ideas and themes contributing to a greater understanding of the potential and complexity of real world research is evident. Capturing this complexity, within Chapter 2 community-based research was framed within a theoretical approach may be most effective in terms of impact and positive outcomes. Two theories were contrasted – one proposing an ecological approach whereby the community is involved in all stages of the research, the other an empowerment approach whereby communities gain access to knowledge, information and resources. The authors concluded that both these theories recognize that in order to conduct good community-based research, the principles of communities as full partners are necessary.

Chapter 3 moved the reader forward with illustrations of the practicalities of supporting such collaborative research and provided the reader with valuable step-by-step guidance on the commissioning of research and the evaluation process. Drawing as it does from practical experience, it added a valuable context to the theory of community partnerships.

The importance of good governance and knowledge of ethical principles was discussed in Chapter 4. The complexity of establishing and consolidating good governance processes across multiple stakeholders, historical and cultural factors and health and social care issues was discussed. The role of the stakeholders and the management of relationships was expanded upon within Chapter 5. Three key perspectives – those of the funder/service provider, the researcher and those communities and settings being researched – were considered. This reminds the reader that close working relationships, collaborations and open communication are essential if the voices of all stakeholders are to be heard and their needs addressed. Building on community strengths and resources allows the research to build upon, and contribute to, the social capital base within the community, contributing to the potential for sustainable prevention and intervention initiatives.

Chapter 6 provided details on real world study designs within the context of the resources available. A key message from this chapter was that a study that is well designed, communicated and meets the needs of the stakeholders is but a first step in a lengthy and complex process, and that a study that is well designed should enable further research and development, thus building on, and contributing to, the social capital base discussed in Chapter 5. Building upon the research design, Chapter 7 discussed the importance of effective fieldwork and what a researcher and the community must consider when they set out to collect data from a community.

In Chapter 8 the evaluation of larger scale and complex community change initiatives, also known as complex or comprehensive community initiatives, was explored. Such initiatives are targeted, place-based collaborative change efforts, which focus on specific areas and target populations rather than on individuals. Given the scale of such initiatives, the authors remind us that more creative approaches to evaluation of these initiatives are required. Authors describe and promote a combined theory of change and a realistic evaluation approach to such initiatives, in order to provide insight to the various stages and implementation of these large-scale endeavours within communities.

The success of community-based prevention and early intervention programmes depends not only on rigorous research and evaluation for evidence of impact, but also on the extent to which the programmes are acceptable to and embedded within the communities of which they are a part. Success depends on the quality of partnerships between the researchers, the commissioners and the community, and requires a careful balance between the demands of rigorous research and the realities of community life. Chapter 9 identified the growing attention being paid to 'secondary dissemination'

(Cohen et al., 2015) of research findings beyond the audience for whom the interventions are designed, the commissioning bodies and/or the funders. Building varied dissemination strategies into research design can, they argued, have significant benefits in that they increase the reach of research and its potential impact beyond the immediate research and practice communities.

But such efforts are not without tension, and require effort in building relationships and maintaining clear channels of communication from research design through to the dissemination programme. Chapter 10 focused on maximizing the impact of knowledge exchange and knowledge brokering and suggested dedicating time and resources to relationship building and iterative consultation to facilitate deeper engagement with the research. Barriers to translating findings and maintaining effective community impact include management structures where partnerships may not be well established at community level, and linguistic and cultural differences, which may need creative solutions to accommodate differing understandings and expectations. This can be particularly difficult when considering time. The time involved in researching effectiveness requires a programme to run its full course before final data collection. This can be difficult for communities to understand, particularly if they are experiencing the positive impact of a programme while it is running. Difficulties can also arise where participants wish to disseminate mid-term data, particularly if it is showing a positive trend. The delay between designing a research study, implementing a programme and being able to report meaningful findings must constitute a key component to be clarified and agreed in effective collaborative research design from the very beginning.

Beyond dissemination in the immediate aftermath of a study, one must also consider archiving research findings, both qualitative and quantitative, for further use. Chapter 11 considered the growing interest and developments in research archiving, paying particular attention to the practical and ethical challenges to be considered. Arguing that it benefits policy, practice and research, the authors suggested that "research commissioners should consider data archiving as a pragmatic solution for ensuring the integrity, accessibility and stewardship of the research they fund...", sentiments which were echoed across the REPP stakeholders.

Key themes and a unified model for communities

Reflecting on the learning and experience contained within this volume and central to the REPP Project, it is striking that the themes reflect the flow of a system in real world research, which contains four crucial elements for success. These can be characterized as the 4Ps: the first P refers to the initial 'partnerships' in service and research design; the second P highlights the significance of the 'processes' that are central to the realizing of the researched intervention in practice with evaluation across time; the third P is the 'product' of the research – the findings in the form of the reports, academic papers and research briefs; and the final P refers to the critical importance of 'promotion' of findings at service, community, local and national level.

Partnerships

Throughout the chapters we have seen the centrality of effective partnerships to the success of the initiative. This is in our view the single key tenet of success across the process, the product and the promotion. Engaging communities in a meaningful way across all aspects of the project from the outset is crucial. An excellent model for this meaningful engagement can be found in Arnstein (1969) and the various applications and developments of this model. Across the engagement process, expectations of deliverables at each stage of the process need to be stated, clarified and managed effectively to avoid disappointments and confusion. The partnership must almost be grounded within a fit for purpose governance structure embedded in ethical principles and practice. As we have seen throughout the chapters, challenges will emerge regardless of the effectiveness of the partnership. These may be within the design stage, or they may be around timing of inputs and outputs, resources, support, training and fieldwork within dynamic communities which may be at risk of being over researched. Without on-going attention to maintaining trusted and effective partnerships, these challenges, as noted across a number of chapters, could cause the initiative to collapse and fail. It is for this reason that *Partnership* is our key tenet within the model.

Process

Process is difficult. The process pathway from start to finish, from commissioning to completion of a child, family or community initiative within a real world context is a complex network of elements and requires a detailed plan. Yet it is also an extremely dynamic journey littered with unanticipated pitfalls and opportunities. A solid partnership will enable the process to stay on track and that strength in the partnership will bring the process back should it lose direction along the way. We have seen earlier that transposing clinical randomized or longitudinal study designs into pragmatic settings is challenging and requires adaptability across a range of stakeholders, given the fluid nature of real world settings. We have also seen how underlying theories may need to be merged to enable realistic evaluations at a population level.

It is also important to recognize when the process is ready to move from one phase to the next and when it is necessary to pause, reflect or recalibrate. Regular communication and trust across all stakeholders is required during the phases of the process. Commissioners must be trusted to commission effectively, researchers to decide the research effectively and communities to engage and communicate their needs and ability to contribute effectively. Comiskey et al. (2015) provide an example of a process evaluation where top-down decision-making and an initial lack of shared understanding impacted upon the implementation of a school-based project.

Product

The final product – the final report evaluating the initiative – is, as we have seen in Chapter 9, merely the first step in the next stage of the full process where dissemination and communication of the findings is crucial. The effective use of the new evidence, be it evidence of success or failure, is essential in the formation of policy, the impact on practice and for further research. Negative findings can be used to inform how the implementation or design of the initiative can be modified to enable possible future success. Positive findings need to be translated for practice or policy. Sustaining a positive initiative needs to be addressed, as does the serious challenge of mainstreaming outside of the original evaluation setting. All of these developments need to be carefully managed to ensure that the original focus and fidelity to the product is not lost when moving from a targeted intervention to a universal one.

As we saw in Chapter 1, the REPP project emerged when a number of researchers involved in different Prevention and Early Intervention Programme (PEIP) evaluations came together to share their experiences. Many of the initiatives informing the chapters in this book have focused on effecting changes at a service level to achieve measurable outcomes for children and families. However, we should not lose sight of the fact that within most community-based research there is a less explicit, and infinitely more difficult to measure, commitment to prevention. This commitment is not focused on changing individual characteristics so much as on impacting on the general health and wellbeing of a group of individuals or a community. While evaluation of the effectiveness of such complex community-based prevention initiatives present many methodological and practical problems (Mercer et al., 2007), reporting findings can contribute to greater understanding of how researchers and communities can work together to prevent difficulties as well as intervene to ameliorate them.

Promotion

Finally, the product must be promoted. From a good research practice and perspective, the importance of wide dissemination and knowledge exchange to different audiences is not only imperative but ethical. Stakeholders working in real life settings have an obligation to ensure the results of the work carried out within a community are fed back to that community and shared with a wider audience as appropriate.

The importance of archiving to ensure the wider accessibility of the data into the future cannot be overstated, especially in the context of over-researched communities. It is imperative that data is used to its full potential and that historical records are maintained. This is all the more important when policy is changed and new evidence is required to be built upon the old. Examples of this might be changes in government policies in the area of pre-school funding or new literacy and numeracy strategies in times of fiscal development or knowing where to make financial savings during economic downturn. If funding cuts or expansion are required, decisions must be based on recent historical evidence and data on what works and what has not worked for whom and where.

Towards a unified REPP model

The four themes evident across this text and the wider work of the REPP Project members can be combined to provide a model of systemic interaction, collaboration and learning for research on children, families and communities within a real world context. In considering the issue of supporting and maintaining quality practice in early childhood settings, the authors of the *CoRe Report* (Urban et al., 2011) highlighted the importance of ensuring that any expectations about change at a service or setting level should be embedded within what the authors called a wider *competent system.* They write that:

> 'Competence' in the early childhood education and care context has to be understood as a characteristic of the entire early childhood system. The *competent system* develops in reciprocal relationships between individuals, teams, institutions and the wider socio-political context. A key feature of a 'competent system' is its support for individuals to realise their capability to develop responsible and responsive practices that respond to the needs of children and families in ever-changing societal contexts.
>
> (2011, p. 21)

When asking what might a 'competent system' for realizing effective research and evaluation in community, health and social care settings look like, we believe that the four themes or 4Ps provide a useful basis for considering the coherence or competence of the overarching system within which the research takes place. To be effective, these 4Ps must be cohesive and connected throughout and beyond the research and evaluation itself. This is particularly important if the effective researched interventions are to be maintained and those that are ineffective reconsidered and changed. Figure 12.1 identifies the elements of the 4Ps REPP model.

In conclusion

Partnerships that are respectful and those that are maintained throughout and beyond the research phase need to be sustained and maintained to continue to progress service/community change. This forms the essential link from *Promotion* back to on-going *Partnership.*

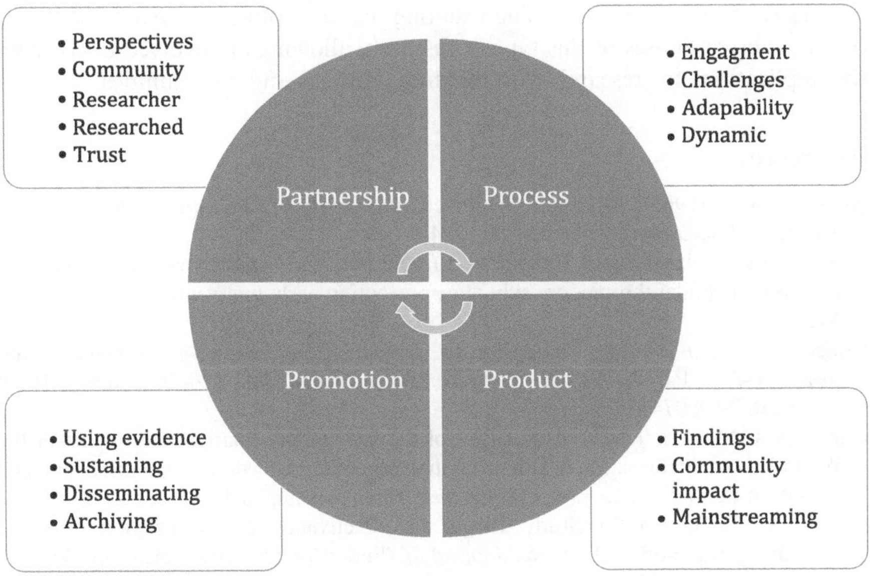

Figure 12.1 Towards a unified 4Ps REPP model

At the *Process* level, account needs to be taken, not only of the immediate research focus, but also of the intervening and often unexpected external impacts on research and service implementation, such as financial crises or policy changes. For instance, how can you factor in the reality of these external factors and their impact on the research, and also reflect on the implications for sustaining the interventions so that they continue to be effective?

At the *Product* level, there is the need to ensure that the language and voice of the findings are appropriate to all those listening – the commissioners, the community, the services and staff and the academic community. Finally, at the *Promotion* level there is a need to consider how to maximize the investment in the researched intervention. Dissemination is one important promotional activity, but there is also a need to close the partnership loop by reflecting on the implications of findings for the services, the community and the local and national policymakers. How can the effective intervention be sustained; how is that monitored? How can the findings be incorporated into national policy for implementation elsewhere? These and further challenges and their prospective and hopefully innovative and novel international solutions we anticipate witnessing in the future.

This book is a collaboration of individual researchers, practitioners and policymakers actively involved in community-based research. The aim was to share their experiences, identify the challenges and opportunities encountered and demonstrate the complexities that emerge at different phases of the process. This final chapter has presented a synthesis of the themes and features of effective community-based research and condensed the key messages from the various sections of the book. The resulting model captures the dynamic nature of the different phases of this type of research, allowing all involved to consider the implications for research with children, families and communities.

References

Arnstein, S.R. (1969) 'A ladder of citizen participation', *Journal of the American Planning Association*, 35(4), pp. 216–224.

The Atlantic Philanthropies Ireland (n.d.) Children and youth page. Available from www.atlanticphilanthropies.org/subtheme/prevention-early-intervention (Accessed 26 May 2017).

Cohen, E.L. *et al.* (2015) 'Designing for dissemination: Lessons in message design from "1–2–3 Pap"', *Health Communication*, 30(2), pp. 196–207. doi:10.1080/10410236.2014.974130

Comiskey, C.M. *et al.* (2015) 'An analysis of the first implementation and impact of the World Health Organisation health promoting school model within urban disadvantaged schools in Ireland', *Vulnerable Children and Youth Studies*, 10(4), pp. 281–293.

Mercer, S.L. *et al.* (2007) 'Study designs for effectiveness and translation research: Identifying trade-offs', *American Journal of Preventive Medicine*, 33(2), pp.139–154.

Urban, M. *et al.* (2011) *Competence requirements in early childhood education and care: Final report*. London and Brussels: European Commission. Directorate General for Education and Culture.

Index